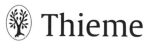

Pocket Atlas of Radiographic Positioning

Including Positioning
for Conventional Angio-
graphy, CT, and MRI

Torsten B. Moeller, MD
Department of Radiology
Caritas Hospital
Dillingen, Germany

Emil Reif, MD
Department of Radiology
Caritas Hospital
Dillingen, Germany

In collaboration with
Eleonore Abel, Dyan Attwood-Wood,
Monika Braun, Beate Hoffmann,
Gregor Hohenberg, Sabine Kadel,
Christiane Koch, Hans Werner Oetjen,
Marcel Paarmann, Christa Riegler

2nd edition

Thieme
Stuttgart · New York

Library of Congress Cataloging-in-Publication Data

Möller, Torsten B.
    [Taschenatlas Einstelltechnik. English]
    Pocket atlas of radiographic positioning: radiographic diagnosis, angiography, CT, MRI/Torsten B. Möller, Emil Reif; in collaboration with Eleonore Abel ... [et al.; translated by Horst N. Bertram and Michael Robertson].—2nd ed.
        p. ; cm.
    Includes bibliographical references and index.
    ISBN 978-3-13-107442-3 (alk. paper)
    1. Radiography, Medical–Positioning–Atlases.
    2. Radiography, Medical–Positioning–Handbooks, manuals, etc. I. Reif, Emil. II. Title.
    [DNLM: 1. Diagnostic Imaging–methods–Handbooks. 2. Posture–Handbooks. WN 39 M726t 2009a]
    RC78.4.M65 2009
    616.07'572–dc22
                        2008043516

1st German edition 1995
1st English edition 1997
1st Japanese edition 1997
1st Spanish edition 1998
1st French edition 1999
2nd German edition 2004
3rd German edition 2004
1st Russian edition 2005
1st Bulgarian edition 2006

This book is an authorized translation of the 4th German edition published and copyrighted in 2009 by Georg Thieme Verlag, Stuttgart, Germany. Title of the German edition: Taschenatlas Einstelltechnik: Röntgendiagnostik, Angiographie, CT, MRT.

Translated by Horst N. Bertram, MD, and Michael Robertson

© 2009 Georg Thieme Verlag
Rüdigerstrasse 14, 70469 Stuttgart, Germany
http://www.thieme.de
Thieme new York, 333 Seventh Avenue, New York, NY 10001, USA
http://www.thieme.com
Cover design: Thieme Publishing Group
Typesetting by Primustype Hurler, Notzingen, Germany
Printed in Germany by Offizin Anderson Nexö, Zwenkau
ISBN 978-3-13-107442-3

Important Note: Medicine is an ever-changing science undergoing continual development. Research and clinical experience are continually expanding our knowledge, in particular our knowledge of proper treatment and drug therapy. Insofar as this book mentions any dosage or application, readers may rest assured that the authors, editors, and publishers have made every effort to ensure that such references are in accordance **with the state of knowledge at the time of production of the book.**

Nevertheless, this does not involve, imply, or express any guarantee or responsibility on the part of the publishers in respect to any dosage instructions and forms of application stated in the book. **Every user is requested to examine carefully** the manufacturer's leaflets accompanying each drug and to check, if necessary in consultation with a physician or specialist, whether the dosage schedules mentioned therein or the contraindications stated by the manufacturer differ from the statements made in the present book. Such examination is particularly important with drugs that are either rarely used or have been newly released on the market. Every dosage schedule or every form of application used is entirely at the user's own risk and responsibility. The authors and publishers request every user to report to the publishers any discrepancies or inaccuracies noticed. If errors in this work are found after publication, errata will be posted at www.thieme.com on the product description page.

For my brother Lars

–Torsten Moeller

For my sister Cornelia

–Emil Reif

Medicine is fortunately in a constant state of flux. New technological developments in particular—for example, in the field of multislice computed tomography—are constantly leading to changes in procedures. In this new edition, we have taken account of this and have completely revised the section on CT. We have also omitted several positioning techniques, such as the intravenous gallbladder examination, as they are no longer up to date, and have included new ones on the basis of the many suggestions that we were delighted to receive from readers of the previous edition.

As always, we have benefited from considerable help in revising the book. Special thanks are due here to the technical assistants in our department, Sabrina Eisenbarth, Anna-M. Kettenis, Lilia Otto, and Andrea Wahl for their resourceful assistance. Our team of authors and experts has also been expanded, and this will certainly have led to a further improvement in quality. We have also made an effort to take account of the relevant guidelines issued by the specialist societies.

We are continuing our efforts to improve this volume even more for later editions and would be most grateful to receive any criticisms and suggestions from readers.

Dillingen, fall 2008
Torsten B. Moeller and
Emil Reif

The book is about radiographic imaging—how to produce images of good quality to provide the diagnostic basis for evaluating and interpreting normal and abnormal or pathological anatomic findings. The arrangement of the material in this *Pocket Atlas of Radiographic Positioning* parallels the arrangement used in the *Pocket Atlas of Radiographic Anatomy,* and in part the arrangement used in the *Pocket Atlas of Cross-Sectional Anatomy* in the same series. This standard arrangement of the content should make it easy for radiologic technologists, as well as physicians with an interest in radiology, to cross-check and compare a correctly exposed radiographic view with normal anatomic findings.

Many good books are available on this topic. What was missing previously was a handy paperback listing at a glance, distinctly, and with a clear arrangement, all the important details that are needed for a good radiographic film—a book that in addition to clearly showing ordinary findings also provides information about variations, offers practical tips and tricks, and presents at a single glance all the criteria needed to produce a well-exposed radiographic image.

More than 200 drawings were also included in order to clarify the essential information for quick reference. The drawings have a two-color design to make them easier to grasp. Details such as projection, central ray, and cassette position are easily seen.

For added clarity, the text is systematically structured into paragraphs describing imaging parameters, positioning and technique, and variations. Where appropriate, tips and tricks are listed separately, as are the criteria for a good radiographic view, which are shown on original radiographs. This presentation should also help direct the attention of less experienced radiologists to the essential information.

We are delighted that some of the best radiologic technologists from various institutions have been willing to collaborate on this project. Their contributions to this book have ensured that there is no undue emphasis on "in-house" techniques from any one institution and that the techniques and variations shown are applicable anywhere. The book includes approaches and techniques used both in Germany and in the English-speaking world, in order to ensure universal applicability. Fruitful and detailed discussions of many issues have certainly also added to the quality and usefulness of this book as a teaching manual for training technologists, and to its value for use in everyday practice.

Extensive collaboration of this kind is unique in the field, and we would therefore like to express our sincere thanks to Dyan Attwood-Wood, Monika Braun, Beate Hoffmann, Sabine Figus, Michaela Knittel, Sabine Mattil, Christa

Riegler, Brigitte Schild, Claudia Zimmer, and Hans Werner Oetjen. Sincere thanks are also due to Drs. Markus Bach, Horst Bertram, Albert Schmitt, Patrick Rosar, Wolfgang Theobald, Stephan Knittel, Beate Hilpert, and Ute Marquardt, and to the radiologic technologists in our own practice for their friendly and knowledgeable critique and advice. Thanks also go to the first author's mother, Friedel Möller, for her support and advice regarding the artistic layout.

Dillingen, August 1996
Torsten B. Moeller and
Emil Reif

Eleonore Abel
Radiologic Tech College
University Hospital Aachen
Aachen, Germany

Dyan Attwood-Wood
Head Radiologic Technologist
Institute of Clinical Radiology
Westphalian Wilhelm University
of Münster
Münster, Germany

Monika Braun
Head Radiologic Technologist
Department of Radiology
Caritas Hospital
Dillingen, Germany

Beate Hoffmann
Head Radiologic Technologist
LETTE-MTA-Training Institute
Berlin, Germany

Gregor Hohenberg, MD
Director, Radiologic Tech College
Saarland University Hospital
Homburg/Saar, Germany

Sabine Kadel
Ludwigshafen Hospital
Medical Tech Training Institute
Ludwigshafen, Germany

Christiane Koch
CT Scan Protocol Designer
Siemens, Inc.
Forchheim, Germany

Hans Werner Oetjen
Head Radiologic Technologist
Editor, *Radiologie-Assistent*
Stadum, Germany

Marcel Paarman
Bad Segeberg, Germany

Christa Riegler
Head Radiologic Technologist
Department of Radiology
Municipal Hospital
Sindelfingen, Germany

Contents

1 Skull

2 Spine

3 Upper Extremity

4   Lower Extremity

Contents

10 Magnetic Resonance Imaging

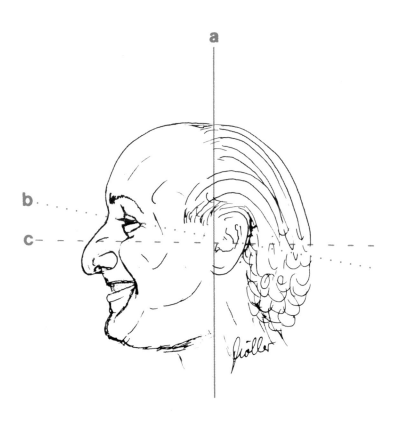

a   Vertical auricular line (connects the two external auditory meatus, divides
    skull into two halves)
b   Eye–ear line (orbitomeatal line, extends from the outer canthus of the
    orbit to the external auditory meatus)
c   Horizontal infraorbitomeatal line (from the bony inferior orbital rim to the
    external auditory meatus)

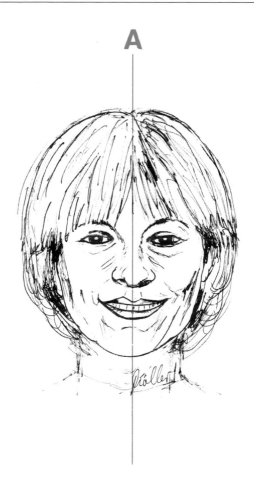

A = Median line

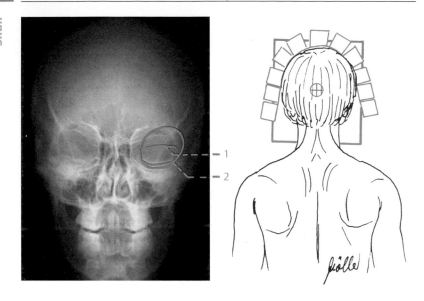

▶ **Criteria for a Good Radiographic View**
- Skull symmetrical and completely visualized
- Skull PA: superior petrous ridge (1) projects into mid-orbit (2)
- Skull AP: superior petrous ridge projects into the lower third of the orbit
- Outer table of the skull visible

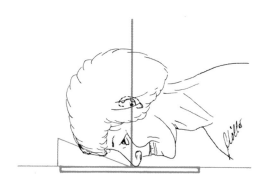

◆ Imaging Technique

Image receiver (e. g., film): size 24×30 cm (10×12"), portrait
Image receiver dosage (sensitivity class): ≤5 µGy (SC 400)
SID: 115 cm (40")
Bucky: yes (under the table, r 8 [12])
Focal spot size: large (focal spot nominal value: 0.6 [≤1.3])
Exposure: 70–85 kV, automatic, center cell

▦ Patient Preparation

–   Remove dentures, glasses; open braids
–   Remove jewelry (necklace, earrings, hairpins, glasses, hearing aid)
–   Open clothes (buttons, zipper)

▲ Positioning

–   Prone, arms along sides of the body
–   Forehead supported on a sponge wedge, tip of the nose rests on the table,
    chin is flexed (horizontal infraorbitomeatal line is vertical)
–   Supine position, head flexed so that the horizontal infraorbitomeatal line
    is vertical, support the head if necessary
–   Tilt tube to align the central ray parallel to the horizontal infraorbitome-
    atal line, median plane in middle of the film, skull straight
–   Head immobilized with weighted band
–   Skull filter, "keyhole," long portion over the region of the cervical spine
–   Gonads shielded (large lead apron)

● Alignment

–   Projection: (1) PA, or (2) AP, perpendicular to the film at the middle of the
    skull
–   Central ray directed to occipital protuberance at the center of the film
–   Centering and collimation, side identification
–   No breathing or swallowing during the exposure

❗ Tips & Tricks

–   The skull is straight when both auditory meatus are projected at the same
    level

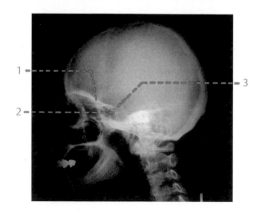

▶ **Criteria for a Good Radiographic View**

- Complete visualization of the entire skull
- Both temporomandibular joints superimposed
- Lesser and greater sphenoid wings of the two sides superimposed (1)
- Sella linear (2) (no double line)
- Clinoid processes superimposed (3)

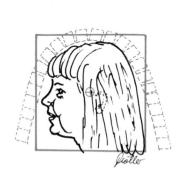

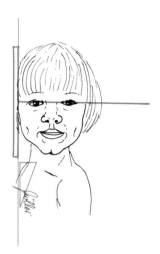

◆ Imaging Technique

Image receiver (e. g., film): size 24×30 cm (10×12"), landscape
Image receiver dosage (sensitivity class): ≤5 µGy (SC 400)
SID: 115 cm (40")
Bucky: yes (under the table, r 8 [12])
Focal spot size: small (focal spot nominal value: 0.6 [≤ 1.3])
Exposure: 70–80 kV, automatic, center cell

▦ Patient Preparation

– Remove dentures, glasses, hearing aids, etc.
– Remove jewelry (necklace, earrings, hairpins)
– Open clothes (buttons, zipper)

▲ Positioning

– Prone (or seated), side of the skull to be examined adjacent to the film
– Upper arm along the side of the body, forearm rests on the table
– Anterior shoulder and chin supported with sponge wedge so that the median plane of the skull is parallel to the film
– Upper border of the cassette 2 FB above the skin line (or simply: middle of the cassette = middle of the skull)
– Skull immobilized with weighted band
– Skull filter
– Gonads shielded (long lead apron)

● Alignment

– Projection: lateral, perpendicular to the film
– Central ray directed to the middle of the skull (about 1 cm above and in front of the external auditory meatus, center of the film)
– Centering and collimation, side identification
– No breathing or swallowing during the exposure

❗ Tips & Tricks

– Put a pillow wedge under the chest of thin patients and children so that the median sagittal plane of the skull is parallel to the table

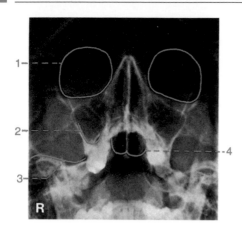

▶ **Criteria for a Good Radiographic View**

− Both orbits symmetrical (1)
− Superior petrous ridges (3) below antral floors (2)
− Sphenoid sinus (4) projected through the open mouth

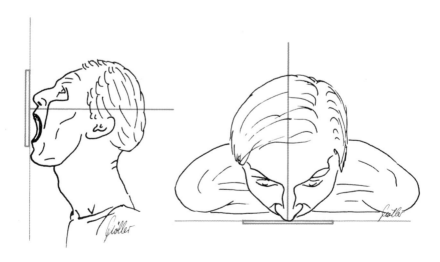

Imaging Technique

ge receiver (e.g., film): size 13×18 cm (5×7") or 18×24 cm (8×10"), por-
t

ge receiver dosage (sensitivity class): ≤5 µGy (SC 400)
: 115 cm (40")
ky: yes (under the table, r 8 [12])
al spot size: small/large (focal spot nominal value: 0.6 [≤1.3])
osure: 70–85 kV, automatic, center cell

Patient Preparation

Remove dentures, glasses; open braids
Remove jewelry (necklace, earrings, hairpins)
Open clothes (buttons, zipper)

Positioning

Facing the film (seated erect)
Head straight (median sagittal plane perpendicular to the table)
Head extended backwards so that the chin touches and the tip of the nose
is about 1 FB from the vertical cassette
Mouth wide open
Extension cone may be used
Gonads shielded (large lead apron)

Alignment

Projection: occipitonasal
Central ray enters 2 FB above occipital protuberance, emerges at the level
of the upper lip (directed at maxillary antrum or inferior orbital rim) in
the center of the film
Centering and collimation, side identification
No breathing or swallowing during the exposure

Tips & Tricks

Before taking the exposure, tape a paper towel to the cassette holder to
put chin and mouth against (hygiene)
If the patient cannot extend the head far enough, have him or her rest it on
the chin and nose, move the tube cephalad and angle the central ray cor-
respondingly, craniocaudad (mostly 12°, but possibly up to 30°)
The cross in the center of the upright Bucky may be used as a centering
aid: center of the cross directly below the nose

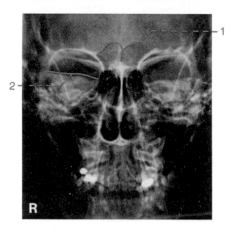

R

▶ **Criteria for a Good Radiographic View**

– Frontal sinuses completely visualized (1)
– Both superior petrous ridges (2) projected over the upper third of the orbit

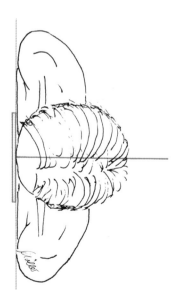
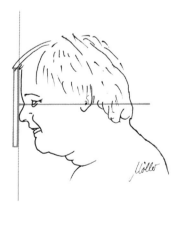

◆ Imaging Technique

Image receiver (e. g., film): size 13 × 18 cm (5 × 7") or 18 × 24 cm (8 × 10"), portrait
Image receiver dosage (sensitivity class): ≤ 5 μGy (SC 400)
SID: 115 cm (40")
Bucky: yes (under the table, r 8 [12])
Focal spot size: large (focal spot nominal value: 0.6 [≤ 1.3])
Exposure: 77 kV, automatic, center cell

■ Patient Preparation

– Remove dentures, glasses; open braids
– Remove jewelry (necklace, earrings, hairpins)
– Open clothes (buttons, zipper)

▲ Positioning

– Facing the film (sitting upright, hands used for support)
– Head straight (median sagittal plane of the skull perpendicular to the film)
– Forehead and tip of the nose resting against the cassette
– Extension cone may be used
– Gonads shielded (long lead apron)

● Alignment

– Projection: occipitonasal, perpendicular to the film
– Central ray directed to the nasion in the center of the film
– Centering and collimation, side identification
– No breathing or swallowing during the exposure

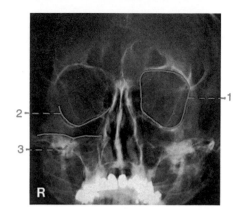

▶ **Criteria for a Good Radiographic View**

– Symmetrical projection of both orbits without superimposition (1)
– Both superior petrous ridges (3) projected below the orbital floors (2)

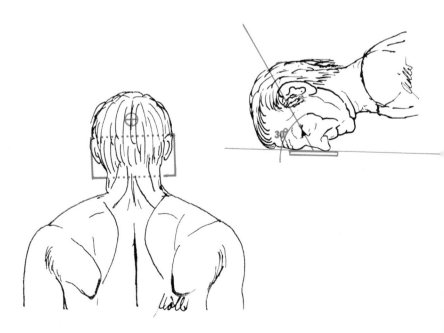

◆ **Imaging Technique**

Image receiver (e.g., film): size 18×24 cm (8×10") or 13×18 cm (5×7"), land-scape

Image receiver dosage (sensitivity class): ≤5 μGy (SC 400)

SID: 115 cm (40")

Bucky: yes (under the table, r 8 [12])

Focal spot size: small (focal spot nominal value: 0.6 [≤1.3])

Exposure: 70–85 kV, automatic, center cell

▨ **Patient Preparation**

– Remove dentures, glasses; open braids

– Remove jewelry (necklace, earrings, hairpins)

– Open clothes (buttons, zipper)

▲ **Positioning**

– Facing the film, prone position, arms along the sides of the body

– Head straight (exactly median), resting on forehead and tip of the nose

– Gonads shielded (large lead apron)

● **Alignment**

– Projection: occipitonasal, 20–30° craniocaudad

– Central ray directed through the median plane to the occiput and nasion in the center of the film

Centering and collimation, side identification

– No breathing or swallowing during the exposure

Skull

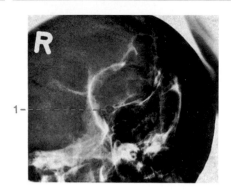

▶ **Criteria for a Good Radiographic View**

– Optic foramen (1) projected clearly into the lower outer quadrant of the orbit

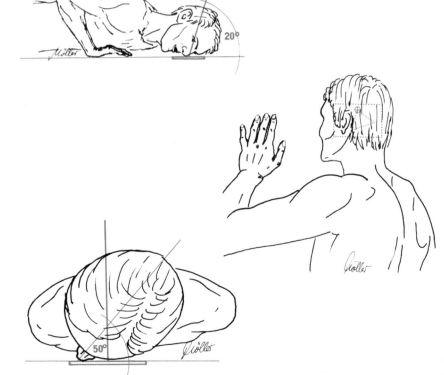

◆ **Imaging Technique**

Image receiver (e.g., film): size 13 × 18 cm (5 × 7"), landscape or portrait
Image receiver dosage (sensitivity class): ≤5 µGy (SC 400)
SID: 115 cm (40")
Bucky: yes (under the table, r8 [12])
Focal spot size: small/large (focal spot nominal value: 0.6 [≤1.3])
Exposure: 70–80 kV, automatic, center cell

▮ **Patient Preparation**

- Remove dentures, glasses; open braids
- Remove jewelry (necklace, earrings, hairpins)
- Open clothes (buttons, zipper)

▲ **Positioning**

- Facing the film (sitting or prone position)
- Tip of the nose and zygomatic arch of the side to be examined resting against the cassette (face turned 50° to the exposed side)
- Orbit in the center of the film
- Gonads shielded (large lead apron)

● **Alignment**

- Projection: occipito-orbital, 5–15° craniocaudad
- Central ray enters at the vertex of an equilateral triangle whose baseline connects the mandibular angle (mastoid process) to the occipital protuberance
- Central ray emerges in the middle of the orbit
- Centering and collimation, side identification
- No breathing or swallowing during the exposure

❗ **Tips & Tricks**

- Always take both sides for comparison

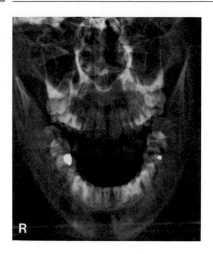

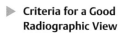

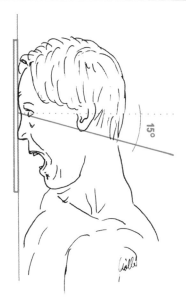

▶ **Criteria for a Good Radiographic View**

– Complete visualization of the lower jaw
– Symmetrical projection of the temporomandibular joints

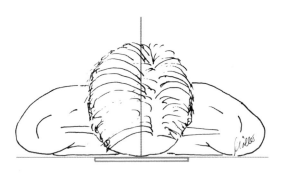

◆ Imaging Technique

Image receiver (e.g., film): size 18×24 cm (8×10"), portrait
Image receiver dosage (sensitivity class): ≤5 μGy (SC 400)
SID: 115 cm (40")
Bucky: yes (under the table, r 8 [12])
Focal spot size: small (focal spot nominal value: 0.6 [≤1.3])
Exposure: 70–80 kV, automatic, center cell

▧ Patient Preparation

– Remove dentures, glasses
– Remove jewelry (necklace, earrings, hairpins)
– Open clothes (buttons, zipper)

▲ Positioning

– A. Patient seated erect (cervical and thoracic spine extended) in front of the upright cassette stand, head straight, chin flexed, forehead and nose resting against the cassette, mouth opened wide
– B. Prone position, forehead and nose resting against the cassette with mouth closed, then mouth opened wide for the exposure
– Gonads shielded (lead apron)

● Alignment

– Projection: occipitomental, 15° caudocranial
– Central ray directed to the nasion
– Centering and collimation, side identification
– No breathing or swallowing during the exposure

❗ Tips & Tricks

– Use a cork to help hold the mouth open
– In the prone position, put a low sponge wedge under the thorax

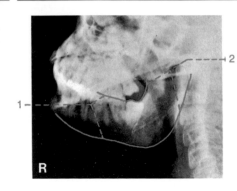

▶ **Criteria for a Good Radiographic View**

- Horizontal (1) and vertical (2) portions of the mandible are shown free of overlying shadows
- The side of the mandible away from the film and the cervical spine are not superimposed

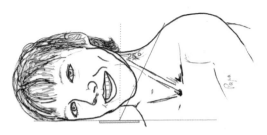

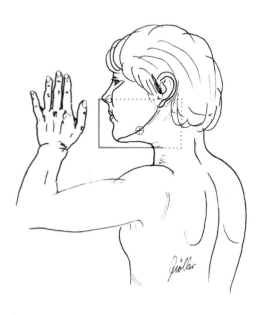

◆ Imaging Technique

Image receiver (e.g., film): size 18×24 cm (8×10"), landscape
Image receiver dosage (sensitivity class): ≤5 µGy (SC 400)
SID: 115 cm (40") or 105 cm (40")   Bucky: no (yes)
Focal spot size: small (focal spot nominal value: 0.6)
Manual exposure: 57 kV; 25 mAs, __ mAs, __ mAs, __ mAs (with Bucky 65–70 kV, automatic, center cell)

■ Patient Preparation

– Remove dentures, glasses
– Remove jewelry (necklace, earrings, hairpins)
– Open clothes (buttons, zipper)

▲ Positioning

– Prone position, or patient seated obliquely in front of the upright cassette stand, head turned sideways, temple of the side to be examined resting against the cassette (median plane of the head at an acute angle to the stand = the mandibular ramus away from the film is projected cephalad out of view)
– Chin pushed forward (to project the mandible away from the spine)
– Gonads shielded (large lead apron)

● Alignment

– Projection: lateral, 25° caudocephalad
– Central ray 1 FB below the mandibular angle of the distant side, directed to the middle of the affected mandibular ramus
– Centering and collimation, side identification
– No breathing or swallowing during the exposure

Variations

1. Mandibular condyles, Schüller position: p. 33
2. Mandibular condyles, Parma position:
   – Head true lateral, median plane parallel to the cassette, affected side placed adjacent to the cassette
   – Projection: lateral, 5° caudocephalad
   – Central ray 2–3 FB anterior to the external auditory meatus, directed to the upper lip and to the temporomandibular joint adjacent to the film, mouth as wide open as possible
3. Patient seated with the affected side toward the vertical Bucky grid
   – Head tilted toward the stand, temple and zygoma resting against the vertical cassette
   – Central ray through the center of the mandibular ramus adjacent to the film (5 cm below the distant mandibular angle)
   – Projection: vertical or 10° caudocephalad

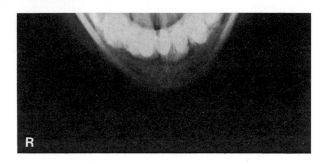

▶ **Criteria for a Good Radiographic View**

– Symmetrical view of chin and lower front teeth

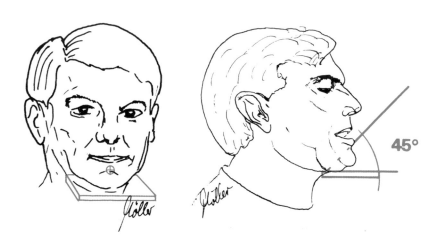

◆ Imaging Technique

Image receiver (e.g., film): size 18×24 cm (8×10"), landscape
Image receiver dosage (sensitivity class): ≤5 µGy (SC 400)
SID: 105 cm (40")
Bucky: no
Focal spot size: small (focal spot nominal value: 0.6)
Manual exposure: 50–55 kV; 20–25 mAs, __ mAs, __ mAs, __ mAs

▨ Patient Preparation

– Remove dentures

▲ Positioning

– Patient sits in front of the examining table
– Cassette raised to chin level (put on a wooden box or patient's adjustable stool lowered)
– Patient extends chin forward as far as possible and rests it parallel to the film in the middle of the cassette (median sagittal plane of the head perpendicular to the film)
– Gonads shielded (large lead apron)

● Alignment

– Projection: oblique, 45°, from cranioventral to caudodorsal (superior anterior to inferior posterior)
– Central ray directed in median plane through the lower lip
– Centering and collimation, side identification
– No breathing or swallowing during the exposure

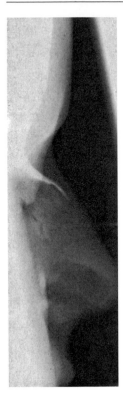

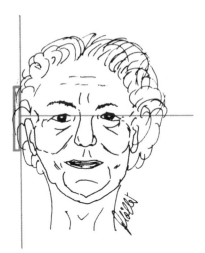

▶ **Criteria for a Good Radiographic View**

- Nasal bones including anterior nasal spine in straight lateral projection

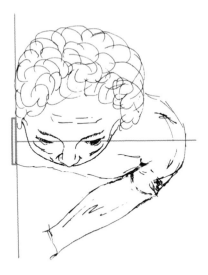

◆ **Imaging Technique**

Image receiver (e.g., film): size 13 × 18 cm (5 × 7"), landscape
Image receiver dosage (sensitivity class): ≤5 µGy (SC 400)
SID: 105 cm (40")
Bucky: no (tabletop exposure)
Focal spot size: small (focal spot nominal value: 0.6)
Manual exposure: 44 kV; 12 mAs, __ mAs, __ mAs, __ mAs

▨ **Patient Preparation**

– Remove glasses and jewelry

▲ **Positioning**

– Patient sits with side to the upright cassette stand or lies recumbent in
  prone or supine position
– Head positioned straight lateral adjacent to the cassette (median sagittal
  plane of the skull parallel to the film)
– Gonads shielded (long lead apron)

● **Alignment**

– Projection: lateral, perpendicular to the film
– Central ray directed to the nasion
– Centering, collimation to the tip of the nose

Variation

Film taken in supine position, head straight, cassette upright on edge

❗ **Tips & Tricks**

– When the film is taken with the patient sitting up, use a head clamp to
  immobilize the occiput

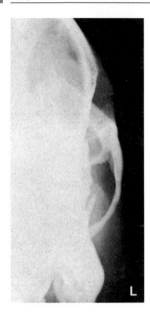

Zygomatic arch, oblique projection

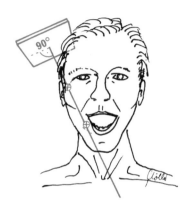

▶ **Criteria for a Good Radiographic View**

– Zygomatic arch projected without any superimposed structures

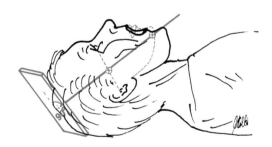

◆ **Imaging Technique**

Image receiver (e.g., film): size 13 × 18 cm (5 × 7"), portrait
Image receiver dosage (sensitivity class): ≤5 µGy (SC 400)
SID: 105 cm (40") or 90 cm (35")
Bucky: no (tabletop exposure)
Focal spot size: small (focal spot nominal value: 0.6 [≤1.3])
Manual exposure: 70 kV; 25 mAs, __ mAs, __ mAs, __ mAs

▦ **Patient Preparation**

– Remove dentures, glasses
– Remove jewelry (necklace, earrings, hairpins)
– Open clothes (buttons, zipper)

▲ **Positioning**

– Supine, arms along the sides of the body
– Head straight, chin slightly extended
– Mouth closed while directing the central ray, opened wide for the exposure
– Head immobilized with weighted band
– Gonads shielded (large lead apron)
– After setting up the projection, cassette is placed behind the head, perpendicular to the central ray, upright and immobilized (with a sandbag or wedge)

● **Alignment**

– Projection: oblique, from ventral–caudal–medial to dorsal–cranial–lateral
– Central ray directed along a line from the middle of the zygomatic arch to the anterior border of the mandible (at the level of the premolar of the adjacent side)
– Centering and collimation, side identification
– No breathing or swallowing, mouth opened wide during the exposure

❗ **Tips & Tricks**

– Middle of the zygomatic arch = midpoint between outer canthus and external auditory meatus

(Continued on p. 26)

Variation

"Jug handle" view (for comparison of zygomatic arches)
- Supine position, head overextended (shoulders supported on sponge pad)
- Projection: submentovertical (ventro-occipital, AP) at 45° angle to the horizontal infraorbitomeatal line
- Central ray 4 cm below mental symphysis (with mouth closed, mouth then opened wide for the exposure), transverse centering through the middle of the zygomatic arch
- Cassette parallel to the X-ray tube and perpendicular to the median plane, behind the head (see above)
- *Tips and tricks.* If there is soft-tissue swelling over the zygomatic region, turn the head slightly toward the swelling

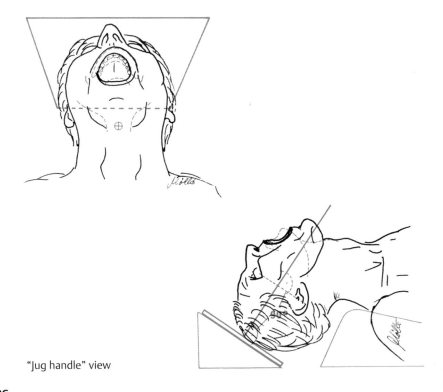

"Jug handle" view

◆ **Imaging Technique**

Image receiver (e.g., film): size 24×30 cm (10×12") or 18×24 cm (8×10"), portrait

Image receiver dosage (sensitivity class): ≤5 µGy (SC 400)

SID: 115 cm (40"); 70 cm (28") also possible

Bucky: yes (under the table, r 8 [12])

Focal spot size: large (focal spot nominal value: 0.6 [≤1.3])

Exposure: 70–85 kV, automatic, center cell

■ **Patient Preparation**

- Remove dentures, glasses; open braids
- Remove jewelry (necklace, earrings, hairpins)
- Open clothes (buttons, zipper)

▲ **Positioning**

- Supine, arms along sides of the body
- Head straight, chin in maximal flexion, head supported with small wedge (orbitomeatal line perpendicular to the table)
- Mouth closed
- Head immobilized with weighted band
- Gonads shielded (lead apron)
- Adjust cassette to central ray (upper cassette border: 3 cm below skin border)

● **Alignment**

- Projection: AP (vertico-occipital)
- Towne: 30° craniocaudad
- Altschul–Uffenforde: 35° craniocaudad
- Central ray directed to hairline (passing through external auditory meatus) and to the foramen magnum, or somewhat above
- Centering and collimation (especially with Altschul), side identification
- No breathing or swallowing during the exposure

Variation

Vertico-occipital projection of the occiput, as in Towne position, but 45° craniocaudad angulation

(Continued on pp. 28, 29)

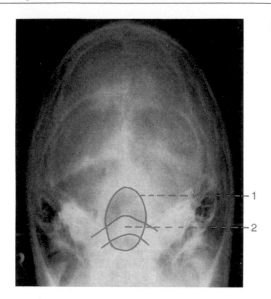

▶ **Criteria for a Good Radiographic View**

Towne:
- Symmetrical, clear view of the occiput (1)
- Posterior arch of atlas (2) projected over the foramen magnum

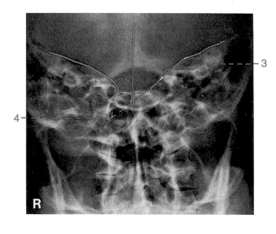

Altschul–Uffenforde:
- Petrous bones and internal auditory canals (3) overlying the orbits
- Symmetrical projection—i.e., tips of the petrous pyramids (4) equidistant to the inner tables of the lateral calvaria

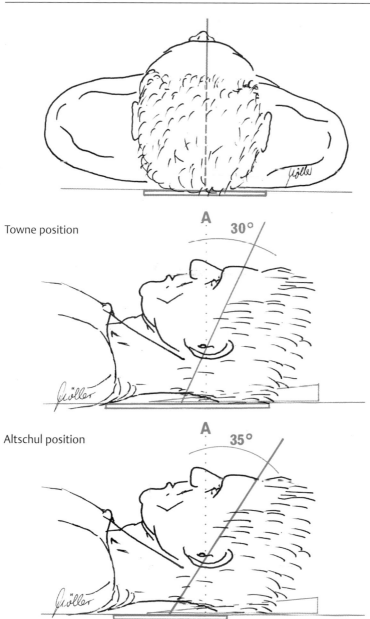

Towne position

A 30°

Altschul position

A 35°

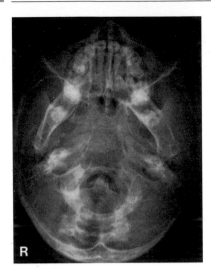

▶ **Criteria for a Good Radiographic View**

– Symmetrical base of the skull
– Mandible projected over frontal sinuses
– Symmetrical view of the mandibular condyles
– Foramen ovale and spinosum are demonstrated

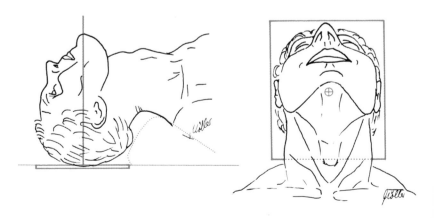

◆ Imaging Technique

Image receiver (e.g., film): size 24×30 cm (10×12"), portrait
Image receiver dosage (sensitivity class): ≤5 µGy (SC 400)
SID: 115 cm (40"), 90–150 cm (35–60")
Bucky: yes (no)
Focal spot size: large (focal spot nominal value: 0.6 [≤1.3])
Exposure: 70–85 kV, automatic, center cell

▨ Patient Preparation

- Remove dentures, glasses
- Remove jewelry (necklace, earrings, hairpins)
- Open clothes (buttons, zipper)

▲ Positioning

- Supine position, either shoulders and back supported (elevated), or patient placed at the end of the Bucky table
- Head extended far back so that vertex rests on the film
- Gonads shielded (lead apron)

● Alignment

- Projection: axial, submentovertical
- Central ray directed to the floor of the mouth at the level of the external auditory meatus, perpendicular to the horizontal infraorbitomeatal line (inferior orbital rim—upper margin of the external auditory meatus)
- If the head cannot be sufficiently extended, compensate by tilting the tube
- Centering and collimation, side identification
- No breathing or swallowing during the exposure

❗ Tips & Tricks

- All preparations, including getting the equipment and cassette ready, should be completed before positioning the patient, as the hyperextension of the head is very uncomfortable; after the film has been taken, the head should be lifted up immediately with both hands and put in a comfortable position
- Extend the head so far back that the shadow of the tip of the nose is projected on the cassette

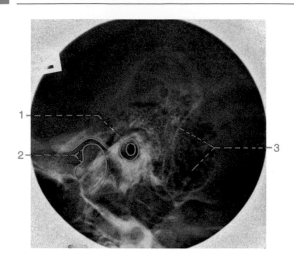

▶ **Criteria for a Good Radiographic View**

- External and internal auditory meatus (1) superimposed as perfectly round openings
- Mandibular condyle and joint fossa sharply defined (2)
- Complete visualization of the mastoid cells (3)

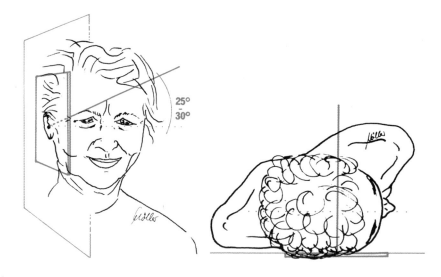

◆ Imaging Technique

Image receiver (e.g., film): size 13 × 18 cm (5 × 7"), portrait/landscape
Image receiver dosage (sensitivity class): ≤5 µGy (SC 400)
SID: 115 cm (40")
Bucky: yes (r 8 12])
Focal spot size: small (focal spot nominal value: 0.6 [≤1.3])
Exposure: 70–80 kV, automatic, center cell

■ Patient Preparation

– Remove dentures, glasses
– Remove jewelry (necklace, earrings, hairpins)

▲ Positioning

– Prone (or anterior oblique) position, side of the skull to be examined adjacent to the film; arm along the side of the body, forearm on the table for support; chin depressed so that the horizontal infraorbitomeatal line is perpendicular to the long axis of the table; anterior shoulder and chin elevated with a wedge until median sagittal plane of the skull is parallel to the film
– The auricle adjacent to the film is folded anteriorly to clearly show the mastoid cells
– Mouth wide open (to demonstrate the tips of the petrous pyramids)
– External auditory meatus on the side adjacent to the film at the center of the cassette, according to the oblique projection
– Head immobilized with weighted band
– May require use of extension cone
– Gonads shielded (large lead apron)

● Alignment

– Projection: lateral, 30° craniocaudad
– Central ray directed to the auditory meatus of the side to be examined (4 FB above the auditory meatus of the healthy side), and middle of the film
– Centering, side identification (for recumbent position)
– No breathing or swallowing during the exposure

Variation

– Schüller technique for the demonstration of the temporomandibular joints
– Schüller variations:
  Rundström projection I—15° tilt instead of 30° (Henschen projection)
  Rundström projection II—35° tilt instead of 30° (Lysholm projection)

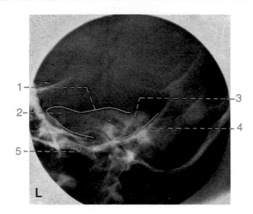

▶ **Criteria for a Good Radiographic View**

- Petrous apices (2) clearly demonstrated
- Crista occipitalis interna (4) lateral to the superior semicircular canal (3)
- Superior petrous ridge horizontal (1)
- Inferior petrous ridge well demarcated (5)
- Mastoid process should be included in the view

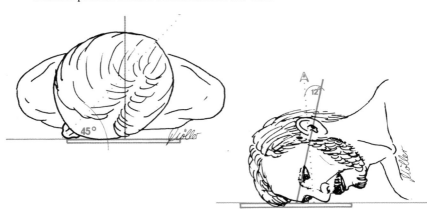

Tips & Tricks

- When positioning the patient, one must watch that the median plane is not tilted. It is therefore best to turn the patient's head from a straight lateral into a 45° position

◆ **Imaging Technique**

Image receiver (e. g., film): size 13 × 18 cm (5 × 7"), landscape
Image receiver dosage (sensitivity class): ≤5 µGy (SC 400)
SID: 115 cm (40")
Bucky: yes (r 8 [12])
Focal spot size: small (focal spot nominal value: 0.6 [≤1.3])
Exposure: 70–80 kV, automatic, center cell (or manual 65–70 kV; 80 mAs,
__ mAs, __ mAs)

▣ **Patient Preparation**

– Remove dentures, glasses; open braids
– Remove jewelry (necklace, earrings, hairpins)
– Open clothes (buttons, zipper)

▲ **Positioning**

Prone position
– Arms along the sides of the body
– Cervical spine straight, chin flexed (orbitomeatal line perpendicular to the
  film)
– Head turned 45° to the healthy side (supported with sponge wedge) =
  zygomatic arch and tip of the nose
Supine position
– Head turned 45° to the healthy side, chin flexed until horizontal infra-
  orbitomeatal line (line A) is perpendicular to the top of the table
– Head immobilized with weighted band (pillow support)
– Gonads shielded (large lead apron)

● **Alignment**

Prone position
– Projection: oblique, 12° craniocaudad
– Central ray directed to the midpoint of a line connecting the external oc-
  cipital protuberance and the mastoid process (about 2 FB medial and 2 FB
  caudal to the protuberance), transverse centering through the external
  auditory meatus of the side adjacent to the film
Supine position
– Projection: oblique, 12° craniocaudad
– Central ray from the midpoint of the orbitomeatal line 1 FB towards the
  orbit
– Centering, collimation, side identification (identify side to be examined,
  reverse mirror view)
  No breathing or swallowing during the exposure

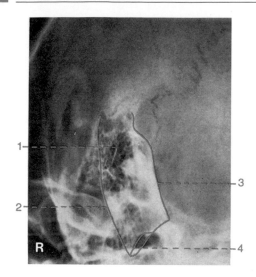

▶ **Criteria for a Good Radiographic View**

– Complete visualization of the petrous bone (along its long axis) from the mastoid cells (1) to the apex (4)
– Long axial projection of the anterior (2) and posterior (3) surfaces
– Structures of the inner ear well exposed

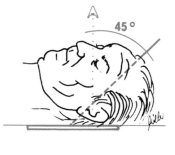

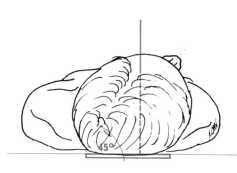

◆ Imaging Technique

Image receiver (e.g., film): size 13 × 18 cm (5 × 7"), portrait
Image receiver dosage (sensitivity class): ≤5 µGy (SC 400)
SID: 115 cm (40")
Bucky: yes (under the table, r 8 [12])
Focal spot size: large (focal spot nominal value: 0.6 [≤1.3])
Exposure: 70–85 kV, automatic, center cell

▦ Patient Preparation

– Remove dentures, glasses
– Remove jewelry (necklace, earrings, hairpins)
– Open clothes (buttons, zipper)

▲ Positioning

– Supine, arms along sides of the body
– Chin depressed
– Head turned 45° to the side to be examined (supported with sponge wedge)
– Head immobilized with weighted band
– Gonads shielded (large lead apron)

● Alignment

– Projection: oblique, 45° craniocaudad angulation to the horizontal infra-orbitomeatal line (A)
– Central ray directed to the hairline at the level of the lateral orbital border (frontal eminence of the distant side directed towards the mastoid process adjacent to the film)
– Centering and collimation, side identification
– No breathing or swallowing during the exposure

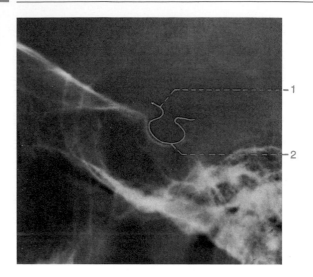

▶ **Criteria for a Good Radiographic View**

– Sella, single contour (no double line) (2)
– Clinoid processes superimposed (1)

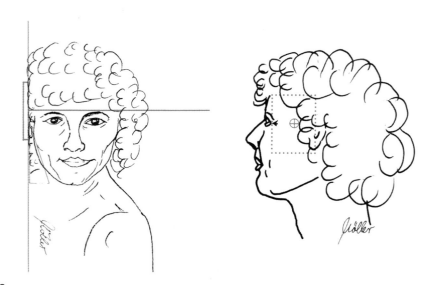

◆ Imaging Technique

Image receiver (e.g., film): size 13 × 18 cm (5 × 7"), landscape
Image receiver dosage (sensitivity class): ≤ 5 μGy (SC 400)
SID: 115 cm (40")
Bucky: yes (under the table, r 8 [12])
Focal spot size: small (focal spot nominal value: 0.6 [≤ 1.3])
Exposure: 70–80 kV, automatic, center cell

▇ Patient Preparation

– Remove jewelry (necklace, earrings, hairpins); take off glasses

▲ Positioning

– Prone (or sitting), head straight lateral, adjacent to the film
– Arm along the side of the body, forearm resting on the table
– Anterior shoulder and chin elevated with a wedge pillow so that the median sagittal plane of the skull is parallel to the plane of the film (back of the head may also be supported with a sponge)
– Head immobilized with weighted headband
– Extension cone may be used
– Gonads shielded (long lead apron)

● Alignment

– Projection: lateral, perpendicular to the film
– Central ray directed to the midpoint of a line that connects the upper corner of the auricle with the outer canthus (2.5 cm above and anterior to the external auditory meatus) in the middle of the film
– Centering, collimation (not smaller than field size), side identification

Variation

Sella: PA projection
– 13 × 18 cm (5 × 7"), portrait; 77 kV; otherwise as above
– Prone position, head rests on forehead, chin slightly flexed, tip of the nose just touches the table
– Projection: vertical, occipitofrontal (PA)
– Central ray directed to the occiput, exits at the root of the nose (nasion), at the middle of the cassette
– Close collimation

❗ Tips & Tricks

– If a lateral skull film was taken, take a film of the sella from the other side, in opposite projection

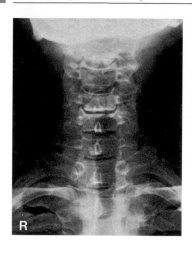

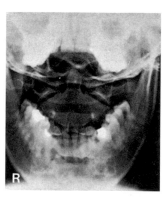

▶ **Criteria for a Good Radiographic View**

– Odontoid process, axis and atlas are clearly visible through the open mouth, occiput does not obscure the odontoid, atlantoaxial and atlanto-occipital articulations are clearly defined
– Cervical vertebrae 3–7 clearly visualized, superior and inferior vertebral plates linear

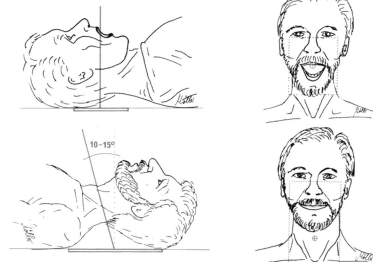

◆ Imaging Technique

Image receiver (e.g., film): size 13 × 18 cm (5 × 7") (odontoid) and 18 × 24 cm
(8 × 10") (cervical spine), portrait
Image receiver dosage (sensitivity class): ≤ 5 µGy (SC 400)
SID: 115 cm (40") or 150 cm (60")
Bucky: yes (r 12 [8])
Focal spot size: small (focal spot nominal value: ≤ 1.3)
Exposure: 65–75 kV, automatic, center cell

▨ Patient Preparation

– Remove dentures, glasses
– Remove jewelry (necklace, earrings, hairpins)
– Open clothes (buttons, zipper)

▲ Positioning

– Supine position
Atlas and odontoid process, AP
– Head flexed until upper teeth (occlusal plane) and occipital bone are
  superimposed (head elevated 15° with sponge wedge)
– Mouth wide open
Cervical spine, AP
– Head reclined so that the line of the mental symphysis—lower border of
  the occipital bone (imaginary line: corner of the mouth—auditory meatus)
  is perpendicular to the horizontal plane of the film
– Mouth closed
– Gonads shielded (lead apron)

● Alignment

Atlas and odontoid process of the axis, AP
– Projection: ventrodorsal, perpendicular to the film
– Central ray in midline at the level of the corners of the mouth
Cervical spine, AP
– Projection: 10–15° craniocaudad
– Central ray directed to the sternal notch and middle of the cassette
– Centering and collimation, side identification

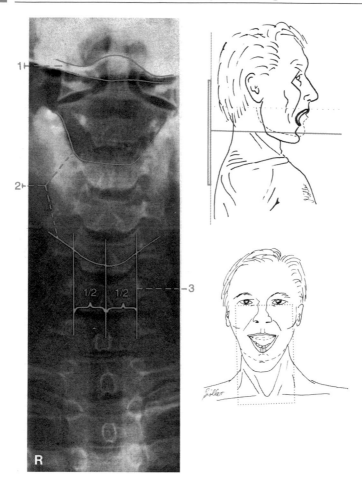

▶ **Criteria for a Good Radiographic View**

– Symmetrical visualization of all seven cervical vertebrae
– Occiput and maxilla superimposed (1)
– Lower jaw is blurred out (2)
– Spinous processes in midline (3)

◆ **Imaging Technique**

Image receiver (e.g., film): size 18×24 cm (8×10") or 24×30 cm (10×12"), portrait
Image receiver dosage (sensitivity class): ≤5 µGy (SC 400)
SID: 115 cm (40")
Bucky: yes (under the table, r 12 [8])
Focal spot size: small (focal spot nominal value: ≤1.3)
Exposure: 55 kV, automatic, center cell
Exposure time at least 3 seconds

▩ **Patient Preparation**

– Remove dentures, glasses
– Remove jewelry (necklace, earrings, hairpins)
– Open clothes (buttons, zipper)

▲ **Positioning**

– Patient sits with his or her back to the upright cassette stand
– Chin flexed (line connecting the occipital protuberance—occlusal plane of the maxilla is horizontal)
– When requested to "open mouth, close mouth; open mouth, close mouth" the patient moves only the lower jaw
– However, head must be held still (head clamp on forehead)
– Upper border of the cassette 1 FB below the corners of the eyes
– Gonads shielded

● **Alignment**

– Projection: ventrodorsal (AP), perpendicular to the film
– Central ray directed to the chin (with mouth closed)
– Centering and collimation, side identification
– Patients may breathe while opening and closing their mouths during the exposure

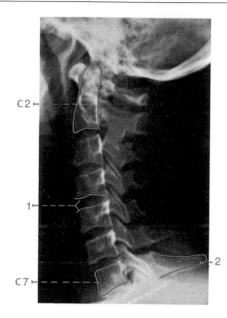

▶ **Criteria for a Good Radiographic View**

....

– All seven cervical vertebrae in straight lateral projection
– Straight projection of superior and inferior plates (especially 4th cervical vertebra) (1)
– Spinous process of the 7th cervical vertebra completely included (2)

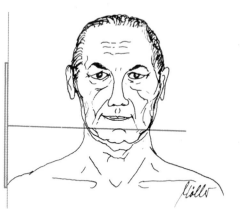

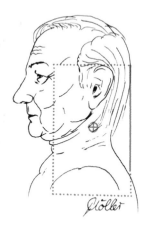

◆ Imaging Technique

Image receiver (e.g., film): size 24×30 cm (10×12") or 18×24 cm (8×10"), portrait
Image receiver dosage (sensitivity class): ≤5 μGy (SC 400)
SID: 115 cm (40") or 150 cm (60")
Bucky: yes (under the table, r 12 [8])
Focal spot size: small (focal spot nominal value: ≤1.3)
Exposure: 65–75 kV, automatic, center cell

▣ Patient Preparation

- Remove dentures, take off glasses
- Remove jewelry (necklace, earrings, hairpins)
- Open clothes (buttons, zipper)

▲ Positioning

- Patient sitting erect, shoulder towards the upright cassette stand
- Head and neck straight lateral (median plane parallel to the film)
- Weights in both hands to pull the shoulders down
- Chin slightly lifted (so that the mandible is not superimposed on the cervical spine)
- Upper cassette border 3 cm above corner of the eye (8×10" cassette at canthus level)
- Gonads shielded

● Alignment

- Projection: lateral, perpendicular to the film
- Central ray directed to the middle of the neck (4th cervical vertebra) and middle of the cassette
- Centering (orbit outside the radiographic field), collimation, side identification
- Breath held after expiration

Variation

- Magnifying view of the cervical spine: like cervical spine, but SID only 80 cm (32")
- Median plane (nose) at mid-distance between film and focal point (at 40 cm) (16")

⎮ Tips & Tricks

- Lower edge of cassette = upper edge of auricle
- Longitudinal centering along the midline of the neck (photocell likewise positioned over the middle of the neck)

Spine

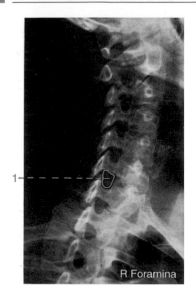

R Foramina

▶ **Criteria for a Good Radiographic View**

– Intervertebral foramina clearly demonstrated (1)

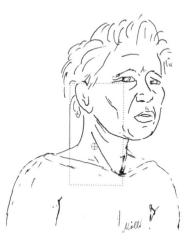

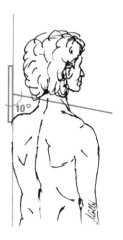

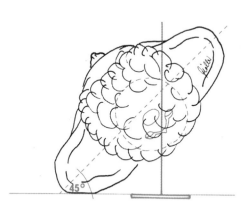

◆ Imaging Technique

Image receiver (e.g., film): size 24×30 cm (10×12") or 18×24 cm (8×10"), portrait
Image receiver dosage (sensitivity class): ≤5 µGy (SC 400)
SID: 115 cm (40") or 150 cm (60")
Bucky: yes (under the table, r 12 [8])
Focal spot size: small (focal spot nominal value: ≤1.3)
Exposure: 65–75 kV, automatic, center cell

▦ Patient Preparation

- Remove dentures
- Remove jewelry (necklace, earrings, hairpins)
- Open clothes (buttons, zipper)
- Hair (braid) combed up or to the side

▲ Positioning

- Patient seated erect, with the back to the upright cassette stand
- One side of the back turned 45° away from the cassette
- Weights in both hands (sandbags) to pull the shoulders down
- Chin slightly lifted (head may be turned slightly towards the plane of the film to get the ramus of the mandible out of the picture)
- Upper border of the cassette = 3 cm above upper border of the ear
- Gonads shielded (small lead apron)

● Alignment

- Projection: ventrodorsal (AP), 10° caudocephalad
- Central ray directed to the middle of the neck (4th cervical vertebra) and middle of the cassette
- Centering and collimation, side identification
- Breath held after expiration

▌ Tips & Tricks

- Magnifying view of the cervical spine: like regular oblique cervical spine, only:
- SID 80 cm (32")
- Median plane (nose) at mid-distance between film and focal point (at about 40 cm)
- Side identification: left shoulder towards the stand = right foramina; right shoulder towards the stand = left foramina

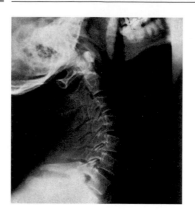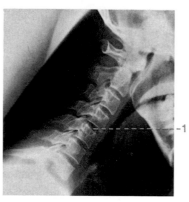

▶ **Criteria for a Good Radiographic View**

– Straight lateral projection of the inferior and superior plates of the 4th cervical vertebra (1)
– All seven cervical vertebrae are shown in maximal flexion and extension

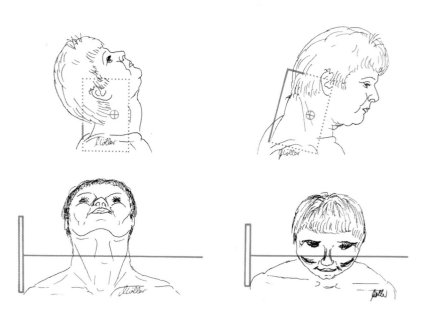

◆ Imaging Technique

Image receiver (e.g., film): size 24×30 cm (10×12"), portrait (extension) and landscape (flexion)
Image receiver dosage (sensitivity class): ≤5 µGy (SC 400)
SID: 115 cm (40"); 150 cm (60")
Bucky: yes (under the table, r 12 [8])
Focal spot size: small (focal spot nominal value: ≤1.3)
Exposure: 65–75 kV, automatic, center cell

▪ Patient Preparation

– Remove dentures
– Remove jewelry (necklace, earrings, hairpins)
– Open clothes (buttons, zipper)

▲ Positioning

– Patient seated erect, shoulder straight lateral to the vertical cassette stand
– Head and neck straight lateral, median plane parallel to the plane of the film
– Weights (sandbags) in both hands to pull down the shoulders (shoulder area may have to be immobilized)
– Head in maximal flexion and extension
– Longitudinal centering (and photocell) adjusted accordingly
– Lower cassette border 3 FB below vertebra prominens (7th cervical vertebra)
– Gonads shielded

● Alignment

– Projection: lateral, perpendicular to the film
– Central ray directed to the middle of the neck (4th cervical vertebra) and middle of the cassette
– Centering, collimation, mark the side adjacent to the film
– Breath held after expiration
– One view each in maximal flexion and extension

❗ Tips & Tricks

– Centering (and photocell) over the middle of the neck
– Always label the films
– To immobilize the head in flexion, use a head clamp for the forehead; in extension, use one for the back of the head

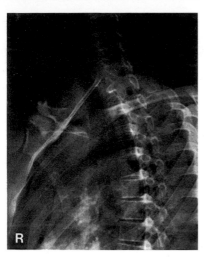

R

▶ **Criteria for a Good Radiographic View**

– Clear demonstration of the 7th cervical to the 3rd thoracic vertebrae in lateral or oblique projection

● **Alignment**

– Projection: lateral or oblique, perpendicular to the film
– Central ray directed to the middle of the cassette
– Centering, collimation, side identification
– Breath held after expiration

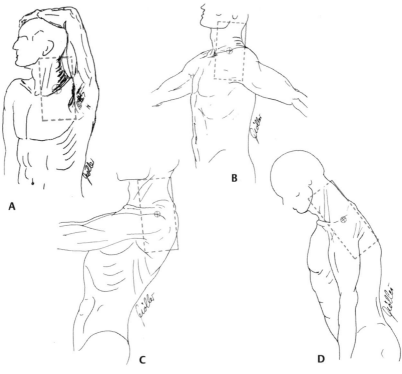

A

B

C

D

◆ **Imaging Technique**

Image receiver (e.g., film): size 18×24 cm (8×10"), portrait
Image receiver dosage (sensitivity class): ≤5 µGy (SC 400), compensating
screen if needed, –/+, minus up
SID: 115 cm (40") or 150 cm (60")
Bucky: yes (under the table, r 12 [8])
Focal spot size: small (focal spot nominal value: ≤1.3)
Exposure: 65–75 kV, automatic, center cell

▨ **Patient Preparation**

- Remove dentures
- Remove jewelry (necklace, earrings, hairpins)
- Open clothes (buttons, zipper)

▲ **Positioning**

A. Oblique
- Patient stands upright with the back to the film, distant side turned 20°
  away from the vertical cassette stand
- The arm away from the film is lifted up, the arm close to the film hangs
  loosely

B. Oblique
- Patient stands upright with one side against the vertical stand
- Arm close to the film is extended forward, the other arm backward
- Have the patient turn the side of the body that is away from the film back
  (about 20°) so that the humeral heads are not superimposed

C. Lateral ("waterskiing position")
- Patient stands straight lateral before the vertical Bucky tray stand
- Patient bends the upper body back (dorsiflexion of the lumbar spine)
- Arms are extended forward (holding on to something in front)
- (Examination can also be done sitting down: both hands grasp the flexed
  knees and pull the shoulders forward)

D. Lateral (bending forward)
- Patient stands straight lateral before the vertical Bucky tray stand
- Patient bends forward with straight back until the head, which is also in-
  clined forward, rests against the headrest
- Both shoulders and arms are dropped forward and down, arms straight
  and turned inward (hands clasped between thighs)
- Upper border of the cassette 2 FB above the 7th cervical vertebra
- Longitudinal centering: (B–D) 3 FB anterior to the spinous processes, (A)
  through the anterior axillary line of the side away from the film
- Gonads shielded

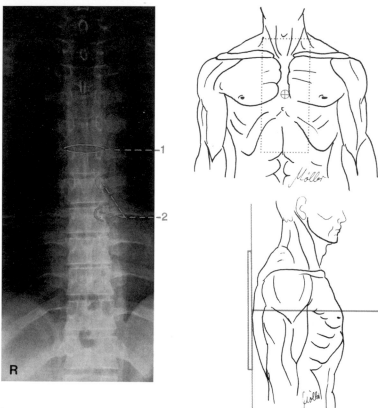

▶ **Criteria for a Good Radiographic View**

– Well-exposed view of all thoracic vertebrae, including cervicothoracic and thoracolumbar junctions, well-demonstrated intervertebral spaces
– Superior and inferior vertebral surfaces clearly delineated (1)
– Costal junctions sharply defined (2)

! Tips & Tricks

– Compensating filter instead of screen
– Centering aid: thoracic inlet (sternal notch) and midepigastrium (solar plexus) palpated with both hands, center = midway between both
– In the supine position, a small bag with rice flour may be placed over the cervicothoracic junction of the spine
– If there is a marked kyphosis present, decrease the focal film distance (more nearly parallel projection due to greater divergence of the beam)

◆ Imaging Technique

Image receiver (e.g., film): size 18×43 cm (7×17") or 20×40 cm (8×16"), portrait
Image receiver dosage (sensitivity class): ≤5 μGy (SC 400), compensating screen if needed, –/+, minus up
SID: 115 cm (40"); 150 cm (60")
Bucky: yes (under the table, r 12 [8])
Focal spot size: large (focal spot nominal value: ≤1.3)
Exposure: 75–85 kV, automatic, center cell

▨ Patient Preparation

- Remove jewelry (necklace)
- Tie braid on top of the head
- Remove clothes from the waist up
- Remove shoes

▲ Positioning

- Patient stands with the back to the cassette stand, arms hang along sides
- Legs are parallel, chin lifted
- Compression band over the lower chest
- Upper border of the cassette at the level of the 6th cervical vertebra (2 FB above 7th vertebra (vertebra prominens), 1 FB above superior shoulder margin
- Gonads shielded

● Alignment

- Projection: ventrodorsal (AP)
- Central ray directed to the middle of the sternum and middle of the cassette
- Centering and collimation, side identification
- Breath held after expiration

Variations

Films taken in supine position
- Legs drawn up, otherwise as above

Thoracolumbar junction
- Image receiver (e.g., film): size 18×24 cm (8×10"), portrait
- Image receiver dosage: ≤5 μGy (SC 400)
- Central ray 1–2 FB below xiphoid process, in midline
- Films taken in supine position (legs drawn up)
- Otherwise as above

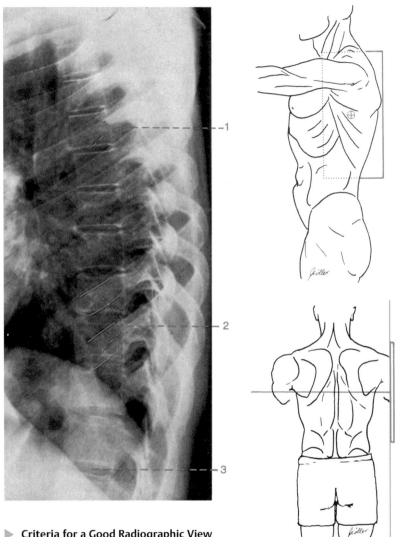

▶ **Criteria for a Good Radiographic View**

– True lateral view with straight margins of the plates of the thoracic vertebrae (1)
– Rib shadows blurred (2)
– All 12 thoracic vertebrae are visualized
– Thoracolumbar junction (3) included in the film

◆ Imaging Technique

Image receiver (e.g., film): size 18×43 cm (7×17") or 20×40 cm (8×16"), portrait

Image receiver dosage (sensitivity class): ≤5 µGy (SC 400), compensating screen if needed, −/+/−

SID: 115 cm (40") or 150 cm (60")

Bucky: yes (under the table, r 12 [8])

Focal spot size: large (focal spot nominal value: ≤1.3)

Exposure: 85 kV, automatic, center cell

■ Patient Preparation

- Remove jewelry (necklace)
- Remove clothes from the waist up, take off shoes

▲ Positioning

- Patient stands with the shoulder towards the cassette stand
- Both legs parallel
- Arms extended forward (holder support) or extended up above the head (patient grasps elbows)
- Upper border of the cassette at the level of the 6th cervical vertebra (2 FB above vertebra prominens) or of the 7th vertebra (vertebra prominens)
- Gonads shielded

● Alignment

- Projection: lateral
- Central ray (a) one hand's breadth anterior to the posterior border of the skin and (b) at the level of the inferior angle of the scapula, directed to the middle of the cassette
- Centering and collimation, side adjacent to the film identified
- No breath-holding; have patient "continue to breathe quietly" during the exposure (ribs are blurred)

Variation

Films taken supine

- Exposure with breathing suspended (to prevent motion on the film)
- Knees flexed, otherwise as above

Thoracolumbar junction, lateral projection

Like recumbent technique, only:

- Image receiver (e.g., film): size 18×24 cm (8×10"), portrait
- Central ray directed 1–2 FB below the xiphoid, and 4 FB anterior to the spinous processes

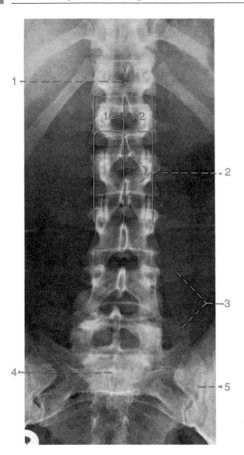

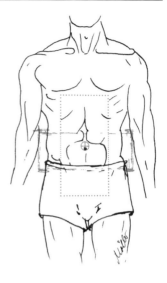

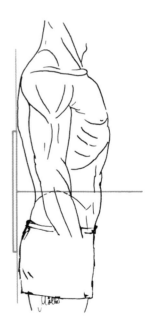

▶ **Criteria for a Good Radiographic View**

– Entire lumbar spine, including T12 (1) and S 1 (4), is on the film
– Spinous processes in midline (2)
– Sacroiliac joints (5) and transverse processes (3) are visible
– On films taken supine: straight projection of the margins of the plates of the lumbar vertebrae

◆ Imaging Technique

Image receiver (e. g., film): size 18×43 cm (7×17") or 20×40 cm (8×16"), portrait

Image receiver dosage (sensitivity class): ≤5 μGy (SC 400)

SID: 115 cm (40") – 150 cm (60")

Bucky: yes (under the table, r 12 [8])

Focal spot size: large (focal spot nominal value: ≤1.3)

Exposure: 75–85 kV, automatic, center cell

▣ Patient Preparation

– Remove all clothes except undergarments

– Remove shoes

▲ Positioning

– Patient stands with the back to the cassette stand, arms hang down

– Legs straight and parallel (if legs are of unequal length, support and build up the shorter leg, and note on the film)

– Compression band across the abdomen

– Middle of the cassette 2 FB above the iliac crest (L4)

– Gonads shielded (testicle cups for men, small lead apron for women, who hold the apron themselves)

– "Erect" (or "supine") should be noted on the cassette in projection onto the abdominal soft tissues alongside the spine

● Alignment

– Projection: ventrodorsal (AP), perpendicular to the film

– Central ray directed to the middle of the cassette

– Centering and collimation (not too close because of the sacroiliac joints), side identification

– Breath held after expiration

Variation

Lumbar spine, AP, supine

– Supine position, legs slightly flexed to reduce the lumbar lordosis, feet set on the table, otherwise as above

Lumbosacral junction, AP projection

– Supine position, hips and knees strongly flexed, feet on the table, thighs slightly abducted

– Image receiver (e. g., film): size 18×24 cm (8×10"), portrait

– Central ray: 3–4 FB below the iliac crest in midline

– Tube may be angled 20° caudocephalad (Barsony technique)

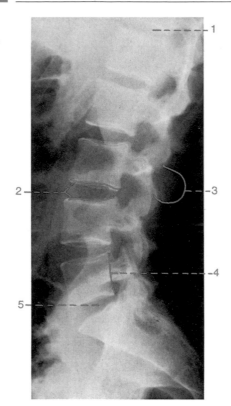

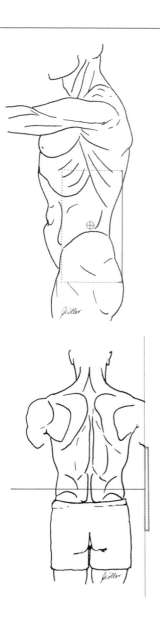

▶ **Criteria for a Good Radiographic View**

- True lateral view with straight projection of the plates of the lumbar vertebral bodies (around the central ray at L3/L4) (2)
- Thoracolumbar (1) and lumbosacral (5) junction well demonstrated
- Spinous processes well visualized (3)
- Posterior border of the vertebral body linear in contour (4)

◆ Imaging Technique

Image receiver (e.g., film): size 18×43 cm (7×17") or 20×40 cm (8×16"), portrait

Image receiver dosage (sensitivity class): ≤5 µGy (SC 400 [SC 800]), compensating screen if needed, –/+, minus up

SID: 115 cm (40") or 150 cm (60")

Bucky: yes (under the table, r 12 [8])

Focal spot size: large (focal spot nominal value: ≤1.3)

Exposure: 85–95 kV, automatic, center cell

■ Patient Preparation

- Remove all clothes except undergarments (take off shoes)

▲ Positioning

- Patient stands with the right shoulder (lateral) towards the cassette stand
- Legs straight and parallel, feet slightly spread
- Arms extended forward (holder support) or extended above the head
- Middle of the cassette 2–3 FB above the level of the iliac crest (L3/L4)
- Gonads shielded for males

● Alignment

- Projection: lateral, perpendicular to the film
- Central ray (a) 2–3 FB above iliac crest, (b) one hand's breadth anterior to the posterior skin border (about midpoint of a line extending from the anterior superior iliac spine to the posterior border of the sacrum, in the middle of the cassette
- Centering and collimation, side adjacent to the film identified
- Breath held after expiration

Variations

Films taken supine

- Legs pulled up (to reduce lordosis), patient put on padding to prevent "sagging" of the lumbar spine (lumbar longitudinal axis), sponge placed between the knees and parallel to the table top to prevent tilting

Lumbar junction, lateral projection

- Transverse centering about 3 FB below pelvic crest, otherwise as above

! Tips & Tricks

- If marked levoscoliosis is present, turn the left shoulder towards the cassette stand

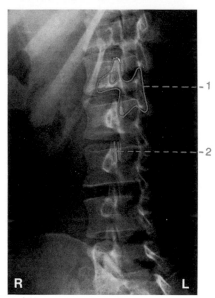

▶ **Criteria for a Good Radiographic View**

– All 5 lumbar vertebrae show the "Scottie dog" sign (1)
– Intervertebral (apophysial) joints clearly demarcated (2)

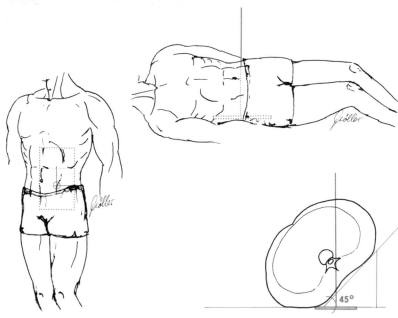

◆ Imaging Technique

Image receiver (e. g., film): size 20×40 cm (8×16"), portrait
Image receiver dosage (sensitivity class): ≤5 µGy (SC 400 [SC 800]), compensating screen if needed SC 400 +/–, plus up
SID: 115 cm (40")
Bucky: yes (under the table, r 12 [8])
Focal spot size: large (focal spot nominal value: ≤1.3)
Exposure: 85–95 kV, automatic, center cell

▉ Patient Preparation

– Remove all clothes, except undergarments

▲ Positioning

– Supine oblique, about 45° (more than 35°, not quite 45°) rotation
– Placed on sponge wedges (one under shoulder blades and one under sacrum to turn the upper trunk into an oblique position)
– Spine extended, legs drawn up to reduce lordosis (knees supported)
– Elevated side of the body straight (median plane parallel to the longitudinal axis of the body)
– Arms extended forward or above the head
– Middle of the cassette 2 FB above pelvic crest (slightly above umbilicus)
– Gonads shielded (for males)

● Alignment

– Projection: oblique ventrodorsal (AP), perpendicular to the cassette
– Central ray (a) 2 FB above pelvic crest and (b) 2 cm medial (towards the umbilicus) of the anterior superior iliac spine of the elevated side (directed to the midpoint of a line from the last rib to the tip of the sternum)
– Centering and collimation, sides marked (R and L to indicate adjacent side of the body and intervertebral [apophysial] joints)
– Breath held after expiration

▌ Tips & Tricks

– For a marked lordosis: adjust the projection 15° caudocephalad

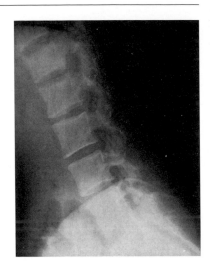

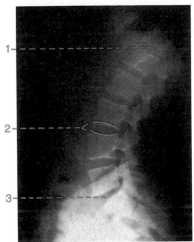

▶ **Criteria for a Good Radiographic View**
- True lateral projection, plates of the vertebral bodies straight (2)
- Visualization of all five lumbar vertebrae, and of the thoracolumbar (1) and lumbosacral (3) junctions

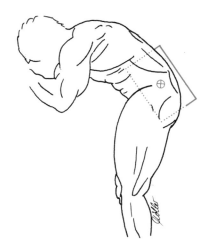

◆ Imaging Technique

Image receiver (e. g., film): size 18 × 43 cm (7 × 17") or 20 × 40 cm (8 × 16"), portrait

Image receiver dosage (sensitivity class): ≤5 µGy (SC 400 [SC 800]), compensating screen if needed SC 400 +/−, plus up

SID: 115 cm (40")

Bucky: yes (under the table, r 12 [8])

Focal spot size: large (focal spot nominal value: ≤1.3)

Exposure: 85–95 kV, automatic, center cell

■ Patient Preparation

– Remove all clothes except undergarments
– Remove shoes

▲ Positioning

– Patient stands straight lateral to the cassette stand
– Legs straight and parallel, feet slightly spread
– Arms extended forward (holder support) or forward over the head
– Maximal flexion and extension
– Middle of the cassette 2 FB above pelvic crest
– Gonads shielded for males

● Alignment

– Projection: lateral, perpendicular to the film
– Central ray (a) 2 FB above pelvic crest and (b) one hand's breadth anterior to the posterior skin border, directed to the middle of the cassette
– Centering and collimation, side adjacent to the film identified
– Breath held after expiration
  One view each in maximal flexion and extension

Variation

– Function studies with left and right lateral bending films (image receiver dosage: ≤5 µGy/SC 400, otherwise as for AP lumbar spine)

! Tips & Tricks

– If there is a marked levoscoliosis, turn left shoulder towards the cassette stand

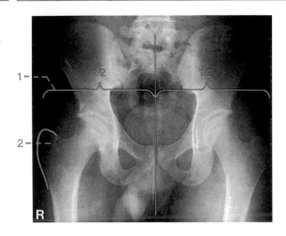

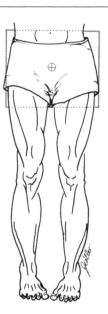

▶ **Criteria for a Good Radiographic View**

– Complete and symmetrical view of the pelvis that includes hip joints, trochanters, and iliac wings (1)
– Lateral cortex of the major trochanters on both sides well delineated (2)

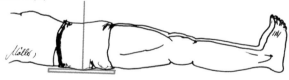

◆ **Imaging Technique**

Image receiver (e.g., film): size 35×43 cm (14×17"), landscape
Image receiver dosage (sensitivity class): ≤5 µGy (SC 400)
SID: 115 cm (40")
Bucky: yes (under the table, r 12 [8])
Focal spot size: large (focal spot nominal value: ≤1.3)
Exposure: 75–90 kV, automatic, both outer or all three photocells

■ **Patient Preparation**

– Remove all clothes except undergarments, remove shoes

▲ **Positioning**

Standing
– Patient stands with the back to the cassette stand, arms are hanging down
– Legs straight, feet slightly turned in (great toes touch, heels about 4 cm apart)

- Adjust any difference in leg length and note on the film
- Compression band across the abdomen (caution: abdominal aortic aneurysm)

Recumbent

- Supine position, legs rotated inward, both knees at the same level (if patient has difficulty straightening one knee, support the opposite side with a sponge pad)
- Upper cassette border 4 cm above pelvic crest
- Gonads shielded for males

● **Alignment**

- Projection: AP, perpendicular to the film
- Central ray directed to the middle of the cassette
- Centering, collimation, side identification
- Breath held after expiration

Variations

Lower pelvic view
- Upper border of the cassette at the level of anterior superior iliac spine, otherwise as above

Pelvis, Pennal I technique
- Projection: craniocaudad 40°
- Central ray at the level of the anterior superior iliac spine, directed to the middle of the cassette

Pelvis, Pennal II technique
- Projection: caudocephalad 40°
- Central ray 4 cm below the upper border of the symphysis, directed to the middle of the cassette

Pelvis, Martius technique
- Position: patient leans in a semisitting/semirecumbent position on the examination table and supports herself with both hands at the sides, with back hollowed; cushion support can be provided
- Radiographic measuring rod should be held transversely over both thighs
- Projection: ventrodorsal, perpendicular to the film
- Central ray: on the mid-symphysis and middle of the cassette

Pelvis, Guttmann technique
- Position: strict right lateral decubitus, hip and knee joints bent
- Radiography scale at the median level between the gluteal fold
- Projection: lateral, perpendicular to the film
- Central ray: 2 FB under the pelvic crest, 3 FB anterior to the line of the spinous process
- Exposure: 115 kV

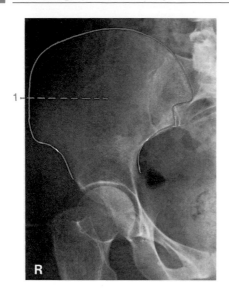

▶ **Criteria for a Good Radiographic View**

– Complete visualization of the iliac wing (1)

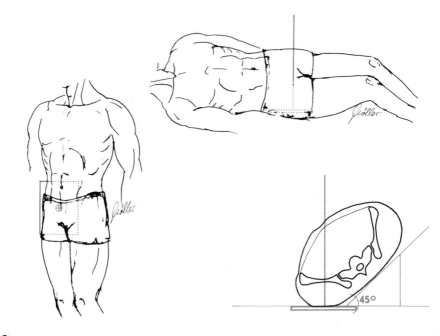

◆ **Imaging Technique**

Image receiver (e. g., film): size 24×30 cm (10×12"), portrait
Image receiver dosage (sensitivity class): ≤5 µGy (SC 400)
SID: 115 cm (40")
Bucky: yes (under the table, r 12 [8])
Focal spot size: large (focal spot nominal value: ≤1.3)
Exposure: 75–90 kV, automatic, center cell

▨ **Patient Preparation**

– Remove all clothes, except undergarments

▲ **Positioning**

– Supine
– Elevate opposite side of the body 45° and support with sponge wedge (leave out gluteal region)
– Affected leg straight, opposite leg flexed (for support)
– Upper cassette border 2–4 cm above the pelvic crest
– Gonads shielded for males

● **Alignment**

– Projection: oblique ventrodorsal (AP), perpendicular to the film
– Central ray directed to the middle of the cassette
– Centering, collimation, side identification

Variations

Low iliac-wing view (for anterior acetabular rim)
– As above, but central ray directed to the middle of the hip joint
Faux-profile view
   Opposite side elevated 65° instead of 45° (for a second plane of the hip joint)
– Central ray directed to the hip joint

❗ **Tips & Tricks**

– *A*lar = Other side *a*lso (for comparison)

Spine

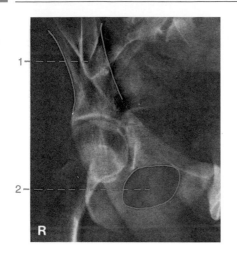

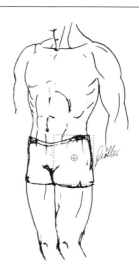

▶ **Criteria for a Good Radiographic View**

- Obturator foramen horizontal–oval (2)
- Iliac wing foreshortened (1)

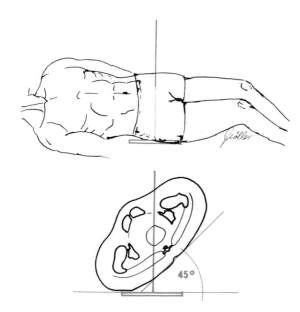

◆ **Imaging Technique**

Image receiver (e. g., film): size 24×30 cm (10×12"), portrait
Image receiver dosage (sensitivity class): ≤5 μGy (SC 400)
SID: 115 cm (40")
Bucky: yes (under the table, r8 [12])
Focal spot size: large (focal spot nominal value: ≤1.3)
Exposure: 70–80 kV, automatic, center cell

▓ **Patient Preparation**

– Remove all clothes, except undergarments

▲ **Positioning**

– Supine
– Elevate side to be examined 45° and support with sponge wedge (under the back, leave out gluteal region)
– Affected leg straight, opposite leg flexed (for support)
– Gonads shielded for males, for females the unaffected side is shielded

● **Alignment**

– Projection: oblique ventrodorsal (AP), perpendicular to the film
– Central ray directed to the middle of the femoral neck = midinguinal area
– Centering, collimation, side identification
– Breath held after expiration

Variation

– High obturator view (at a second plane of the iliac wing = alar view): central ray directed to the middle of the iliac wing, otherwise as above.

❗ **Tips & Tricks**

– "*Up*turator" view: side to be examined *up*
– By using a larger film and centering over the midpelvis, one also gets a view of the opposite side (when looking for a fracture of the pelvic ring, for example)

Spine

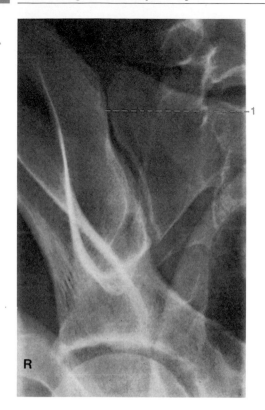

R

▶ **Criteria for a Good Radiographic View**

– Unobstructed projection of the sacroiliac joints (1)

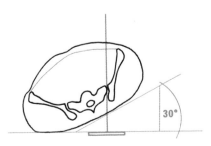

30°

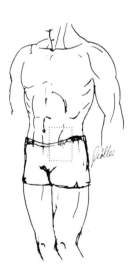

◆ Imaging Technique

Image receiver (e.g., film): size 18×24cm (8×10"), portrait
Image receiver dosage (sensitivity class): ≤5 µGy (SC 400)
SID: 115cm (40")
Bucky: yes (under the table, r 12 [8])
Focal spot size: large (focal spot nominal value: ≤1.3)
Exposure: 75–90 kV, automatic, center cell

▮ Patient Preparation

- Remove all clothes, except undergarments
- Evacuate bowel (enema if needed)

▲ Positioning

- Supine position
- Elevate side to be examined 30–45°
- Gonads shielded for males
- Middle of the cassette 2–3 FB below pelvic crest

● Alignment

- Projection: oblique ventrodorsal (AP), perpendicular to the middle of the cassette
- Central ray 3 FB medial to the anterior superior iliac spine
  Centering, collimation, side identification
- Breath held after expiration

▮ Tips & Tricks

- Take views of both sides for comparison

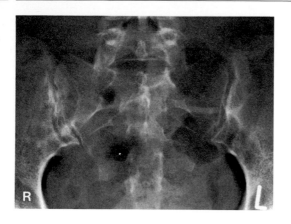

▶ **Criteria for a Good Radiographic View**
– Complete visualization of the sacroiliac joints

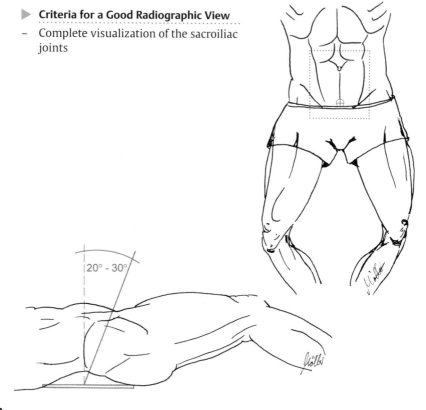

20° - 30°

◆ Imaging Technique

Image receiver (e.g., film): size 24×30 cm (10×12"), portrait 18×24 cm (or 8×10", landscape)
Image receiver dosage (sensitivity class): ≤5 µGy (SC 400)
SID: 115 cm (40")
Bucky: yes (r 12 [8])
Focal spot size: large (focal spot nominal value: ≤1.3)
Manual exposure: 75–90 kV; __ mAs, __ mAs, __ mAs

▦ Patient Preparation

- Remove all clothes, except undergarments
- Evacuate bowel (enema if needed)

▲ Positioning

- Supine, arms along the sides of the body
- Hips and knee joints flexed and abducted
- Gonads shielded for males
- Middle of the cassette 2–3 FB below pelvic crest

● Alignment

- Projection: ventrodorsal (AP), 20–30° caudocephalad (or vertical)
- Central ray 2 FB above the border of the symphysis
- Centering, collimation, side identification
- Breath held after expiration

Variation

Lithotomy position
- Patient draws up both legs (to reduce lordosis) and abducts the flexed legs
- Central ray vertical

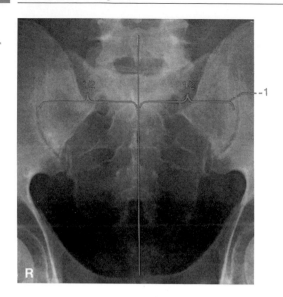

▶ **Criteria for a Good Radiographic View**
....

–   Unobstructed, unforeshortened, and symmetrical (1) view of the sacrum, sacroiliac joints, and the 5th lumbar vertebra

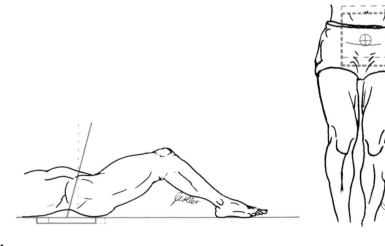

◆ **Imaging Technique**

Image receiver (e.g., film): size 24×30 cm (10×12"), portrait
Image receiver dosage (sensitivity class): ≤5 µGy (SC 400)
SID: 115 cm (40")
Bucky: yes (under the table, r 12 [8])
Focal spot size: large (focal spot nominal value: ≤1.3)
Exposure: 75–90 kV, automatic, center cell

■ **Patient Preparation**

- Remove all clothes, except undergarments
- Evacuate bowel (enema if needed)

▲ **Positioning**

- Supine, arms along the sides of the body
- Hip and knee joints flexed (sponge support under knees)
- Gonads shielded for males
- Middle of the cassette at the level of the anterior superior iliac spine in median plane (lower cassette border at the level of the symphysis, upper cassette border at pelvic crest)

● **Alignment**

- Projection: ventrodorsal (AP), 20° caudocephalad (or vertical)
- Central ray 2 FB above border of the symphysis (or, in vertical projection, medial plane at the level of the anterior superior iliac spine), directed to the middle of the cassette
- Centering, collimation, side identification
- Breath held after expiration

Variation

Coccyx, AP projection
- Projection: 20° craniocaudad
- Central ray a hand's breadth above the symphysis, directed to the middle of the cassette
- Exposure: 76 kV, automatic, center cell
- Otherwise as above

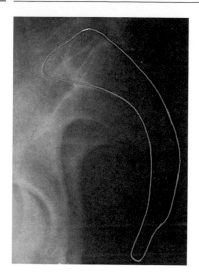

▶ **Criteria for a Good Radiographic View**

– Lateral view shows straight and complete visualization of sacrum and coccyx

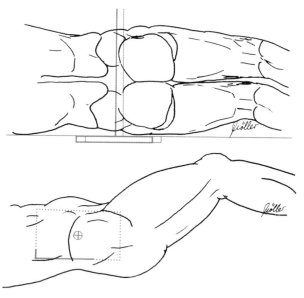

◆ Imaging Technique

Image receiver (e.g., film): size 20×40 cm (8×16") or 24×30 cm (10×12"), portrait
Image receiver dosage (sensitivity class): $\leq 5\,\mu$Gy (SC 400 [SC 800])
SID: 115 cm (40")
Bucky: yes (under the table, r 12)
Focal spot size: large (focal spot nominal value: ≤ 1.3)
Exposure: 80–90 kV, automatic, center cell (density compensation + 1)

■ Patient Preparation

– Remove all clothes, except undergarments

▲ Positioning

– Straight lateral position, hips and knee joints flexed
– Sponge padding under waist and knees
– Middle of the cassette:
– Sacrum: midpoint between pelvic crest and tip of the coccyx
– Coccyx: over the lower third between pelvic crest and tip of the coccyx
– Sacrum and coccyx: a hand's breadth below the pelvic crest and a hand's breadth anterior to the posterior skin border (more anterior in obese patients)
– Gonads shielded for males

● Alignment

– Projection: lateral, perpendicular to the film
– Central ray directed to the middle of the cassette (nearly one hand's breadth below the pelvic crest for the sacrum, more for the coccyx)
– Centering, collimation (identify side adjacent to the film)
– Breath held after expiration

❗ Tips & Tricks

– Extension cone may be used (less overexposure)

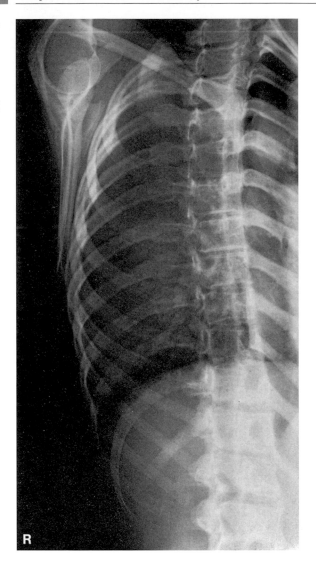

▶ **Criteria for a Good Radiographic View**

– Ribs well exposed and completely visualized

◆ **Imaging Technique**

Image receiver (e.g., film): size 35×43 cm (14×17") (or 18×43 cm [7×17"] for oblique), portrait

Image receiver dosage (sensitivity class): ≤5 µGy (SC 400), use of compensating screen possible, –/+, minus up

SID: 115 cm (40")

Bucky: yes (under the table, r 8 [12])

Focal spot size: large (focal spot nominal value: ≤1.3)

Exposure: 60–65 kV or 70–75 kV (for lower ribs), automatic, center cell

■ **Patient Preparation**

– Remove all clothes from the waist up
– Remove jewelry (necklace, earrings)
– Have hair tied up on top of the head

▲ **Positioning**

The injured part of the rib is always placed closest to the film:

– A. Patient stands/lies with his back (or, depending on the injury, with his chest) straight against the cassette
– Head turned to the healthy side
– Arms along the sides of the body, slightly rotated inward and abducted (hands on hips)
– Upper border of the cassette at the level the 6th cervical vertebra (above vertebra prominens) (or lower border of the cassette 2 cm above pelvic crest)
– B. Healthy side turned up 30–40°, affected side next to the film (prone or supine position)
– Gonads shielded (short lead apron)

● **Alignment**

– Projection: perpendicular (AP or PA) to the film
– Central ray directed to the middle of the film
– Centering, collimation, side identification
– Breathing suspended after inspiration

(Continued on pp. 80, 81)

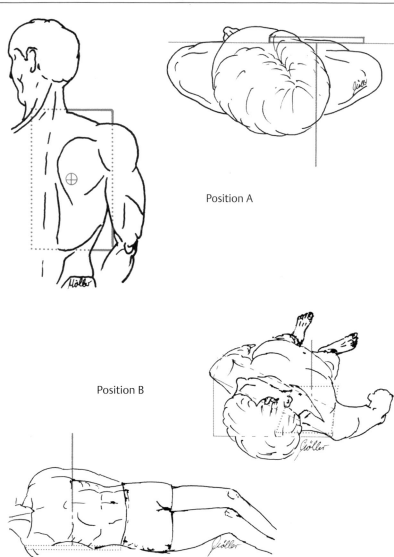

Position A

Position B

Variation

- Additional views of the lower ribs:
- Image receiver (e.g., film): size 24×30 cm (10×12"), portrait
- Supine position, healthy side elevated 45°, arms turned up
- Lower cassette border 2 FB above pelvic crest
- Breath held in expiration (diaphragms elevated: photocell over the upper abdomen = good exposure of the lower ribs)

! Tips & Tricks

- Mark the area that hurts

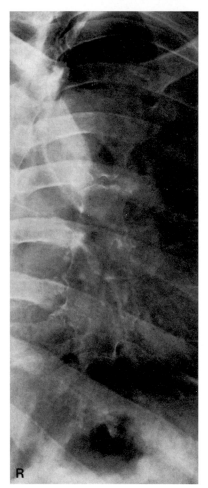

R

▶ **Criteria for a Good Radiographic View**

– Sternum clearly demonstrated (thoracic spine or scapula not superimposed)

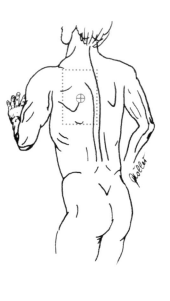

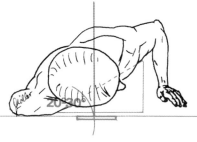

20–30°

◆ Imaging Technique

Image receiver (e.g., film): size 24×30 cm (10×12"), portrait
Image receiver dosage (sensitivity class): ≤5 µGy (SC 400)
SID: 115 cm (40")
Bucky: yes (under the table, r 8 [12])
Focal spot size: large (focal spot nominal value: ≤1.3)
Exposure: 60–74 kV, automatic, center cell

▩ Patient Preparation

– Remove all clothes from the waist up
– Remove jewelry (necklace, earrings)
– Have hair tied up on top of the head

▲ Positioning

– Prone, left (right) side turned up about 15° (–30°), to move sternum away from the overlying thoracic spine, and supported with the left (right) hand
– Wedge pad for additional support
– Other arm along the side of the body
– Upper cassette border 2 FB above jugular fossa
– Gonads shielded (small lead apron)

● Alignment

– Projection: dorsoventral (PA), perpendicular to the film
– Central ray 3 FB left (right) of the thoracic spine (at about the level of the medial scapular border on the elevated side) directed to the middle of the film
– Centering, collimation, side identification
– Breath held after expiration

❗ Tips & Tricks

– Small patient = elevate more
– Large patient = elevate less

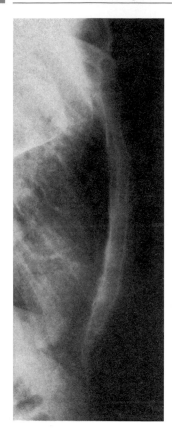

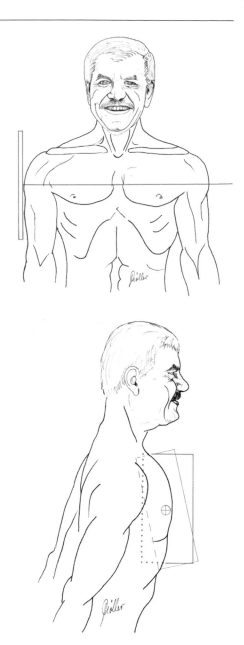

▶ **Criteria for a Good Radiographic View**

– Complete visualization of the sternum

◆ Imaging Technique

Image receiver (e.g., film): size 24×30 cm (10×12") or 30×40 cm (12×16"), portrait
Image receiver dosage (sensitivity class): ≤5 µGy (SC 400)
SID: 115 cm (40")
Bucky: yes (under the table, r 8 [12])
Focal spot size: small (focal spot nominal value ≤1.3)
Exposure: 60–75 kV, automatic, center cell

▦ Patient Preparation

- Remove jewelry (necklace)
- Remove all clothes from the waist up

▲ Positioning

- Patient stands with shoulder lateral to the vertical cassette stand
- Arms behind the back
- Chest pushed forward
- Upper border of the cassette 3 cm above the sternal notch
- Gonads shielded

● Alignment

- Projection: lateral
- Central ray to the middle of the sternum and middle of the cassette (about 2 FB behind the anterior surface)
- Centering, collimation (place the cassette obliquely, if possible, to collimate narrowly)
- Breathing suspended in inspiration

Variation

- Lateral sternum in the recumbent position: supine, either arms extended upward or back supported with pillows with arms hanging down over the sides
- Cassettes placed upright against the side

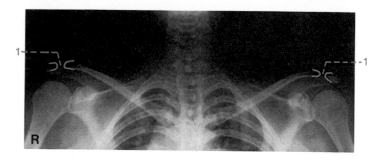

▶ **Criteria for a Good Radiographic View**

– Complete visualization of both acromioclavicular joints (1)

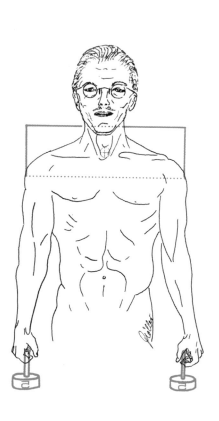

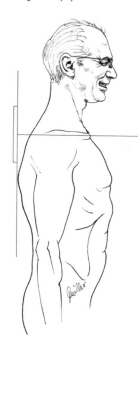

◆ **Imaging Technique**

Image receiver (e.g., film): size 20×60 cm (8×24"), landscape (or larger size, collimated)

Image receiver dosage (sensitivity class): ≤5 µGy (SC 400)

SID: 115 cm (40"), up to 150 cm (60")

Bucky: no (tabletop exposure)

Focal spot size: small (focal spot nominal value ≤1.3)

Manual exposure: 60–75 kV; 10–16 mAs, __ mAs, __ mAs, __ mAs

▦ **Patient Preparation**

– Remove jewelry (necklace, earrings)
– Remove all clothes from the waist up

▲ **Positioning**

– Patient with the back to the vertical cassette stand, shoulders pulled back, chest pushed out
– Arms hang along the sides of the body
– Weights (about 5–10 kg) in both hands
– Upper cassette border 2 cm above the superior margin of the shoulder
– Gonads shielded (lead apron)

● **Alignment**

– Projection: ventrodorsal (AP), perpendicular to the film
– Central ray directed to the sternal notch and middle of the cassette; the (horizontal) transverse center passes through both acromioclavicular joints
– Centering, collimation, sides identified; "weight-bearing, bilateral, 5 kg" noted on the film
– Breath held after expiration

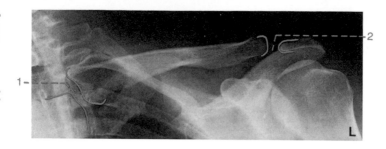

▶ **Criteria for a Good Radiographic View**

– Complete visualization of the clavicle, including the sternoclavicular (1) and acromioclavicular joint (2)

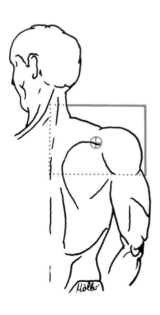
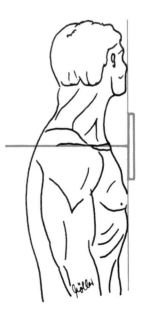

◆ **Imaging Technique**

Image receiver (e. g., film): size 24×30 cm (10×12") or 18×24 cm (8×10"), landscape
Image receiver dosage (sensitivity class): ≤5 µGy (SC 400)
SID: 115 cm (40")
Bucky: yes (under the table, r 8 [12])
Focal spot size: small (focal spot nominal value ≤1.3)
Exposure: 60–75 kV, automatic, center cell (manual: 60–74 kV; 16–20 mAs, __ mAs, __ mAs)

■ **Patient Preparation**

– Remove jewelry (necklace, earrings)
– Remove all clothes from the waist up

▲ **Positioning**

– Patient stands with the chest to the cassette stand, clavicle placed against the film (or supine position)
– Face turned to the opposite side
– Arm on the side to be examined rotated inward (back of the hand towards the stand)
– Upper cassette border 2 FB above shoulder level
– Gonads shielded (lead apron over the back)

● **Alignment**

– Projection: dorsoventral (PA), perpendicular to the film
– Central ray directed to the midpoint of the clavicle and middle of the film
– Centering, collimation, side identification
– Breathing suspended in expiration

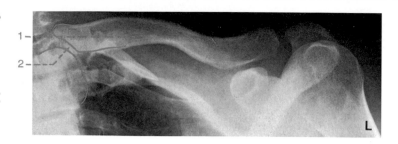

▶ **Criteria for a Good Radiographic View**
....
- Visualization of the entire clavicle (1)
- Middle and lateral portions without superimposed shadows (with the exception of the sternoclavicular joint [2])

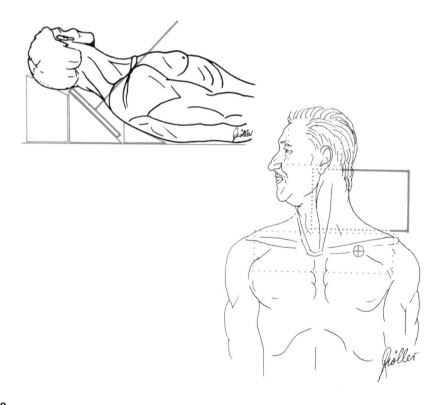

Upper Extremity

◆ **Imaging Technique**

Image receiver (e.g., film): size 24×30 cm (10×12") or 18×24 cm (8×10"), landscape
Image receiver dosage (sensitivity class): ≤5 µGy (SC 400)
SID: 105 cm (40")
Bucky: no (tabletop technique)
Focal spot size: small (focal spot nominal value ≤1.3)
Manual exposure: 60 (–75) kV; 10 mAs, __ mAs, __ mAs

■ **Patient Preparation**

- Remove jewelry (necklace, earrings)
- Remove all clothes from the waist up

▲ **Positioning**

- Supine position, arms along the sides of the body, head turned to the opposite side
- Shoulder and head slightly elevated and supported with sponge pad
- Cassette placed against the back of the shoulder at an oblique angle of about 45° to the tabletop (and supported with a wedge, additional sandbag if needed)
- Gonads shielded (lead apron)

● **Alignment**

- Projection: 45° cephalad angulation (oblique ventrocaudad to dorsocephalad [oblique AP]) perpendicular to the film
- Central ray directed to the midpoint of the clavicle and middle of the film
- Centering, collimation, side identification
- Breath held after expiration

Variation

- Patient in supine position (or stands with the back to the vertical grid)
- Healthy shoulder slightly elevated (supported) until clavicle is parallel to the cassette
- Hand on the side to be examined is supinated
- Projection: 30° caudocephalad
- Central ray directed to the midpoint of the clavicle and the middle of the film
- Exposure: 55 kV, automatic, center cell

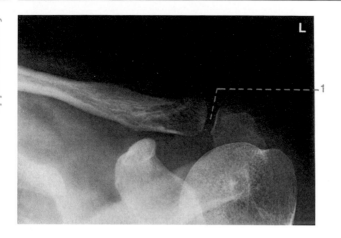

▶ **Criteria for a Good Radiographic View**

– Unobstructed view of the acromioclavicular joint (1)

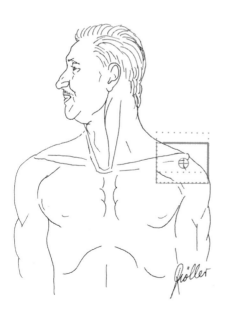

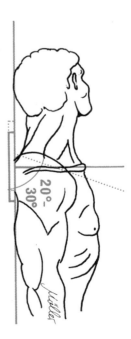

◆ **Imaging Technique**

Image receiver (e. g., film): size 18 × 24 cm (8 × 10") or 13 × 18 cm (5 × 7"), land-scape

Image receiver dosage (sensitivity class): ≤ 5 µGy (SC 400)

SID: 115 cm (40") or 105 cm (40")

Bucky: yes (no), under the table (tabletop)

Focal spot size: small (focal spot nominal value ≤ 1.3)

Exposure: 60 (–75) kV, automatic, center cell (manual: 60 (–75) kV, 10 mAs, __ mAs, __ mAs)

▨ **Patient Preparation**

– Remove jewelry (necklace)
– Remove all clothes from the waist up

▲ **Positioning**

– Patient sitting or lying with the back to the film
– Arms along the sides of the body, inside of the hand turned out
– Upper cassette border 2 FB above the superior margin of the shoulder in vertical projection, higher if the tube is angled
– Gonads shielded (lead apron)

● **Alignment**

– Projection: ventrodorsal (AP), perpendicular to the film (perhaps 20–35° caudocephalad)
– Central ray directed to the acromioclavicular joint
– Centering, collimation, side identification
– Breath held after expiration

❗ **Tips & Tricks**

– This view is also taken as a 3 rd view of the shoulder joint (see p. 101)
– A compensating filter may be used if available

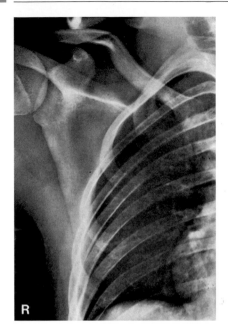

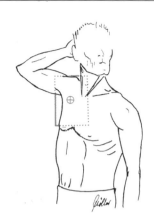

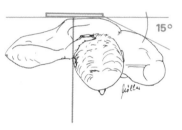

▶ Criteria for a Good Radiographic View

– Complete visualization of the scapula, no ribs overlying the lateral portion

Position A

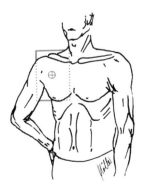

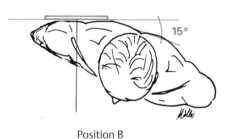

Position B

◆ **Imaging Technique**

Image receiver (e.g., film): size 24×30 cm (10×12"), portrait
Image receiver dosage (sensitivity class): ≤5 µGy (SC 400)
SID: 115 cm (40")
Bucky: yes (vertical Bucky grid, r 8 [12])
Focal spot size: small (focal spot nominal value ≤1.3)
Exposure: 60–75 kV, automatic, center cell

▦ **Patient Preparation**

– Remove jewelry (necklace, earrings)
– Remove all clothes from the waist up

▲ **Positioning**

– Patient with the back and scapula flat against the upright cassette stand
– The unaffected side is elevated 15° (scapula parallel to the film)
– Chin lifted, head turned to the opposite side
– Hand on the affected side turned up and put on top of the head (A), or placed on the hip (arm abducted, B)
– Upper cassette border at the level of the superior border of the shoulder
– Gonads shielded (small lead apron)

● **Alignment**

– Projection: ventrodorsal (AP), perpendicular to the film
– Central ray directed to the midpoint of the scapula and middle of the film
– Centering, collimation, side identification
– Breathing suspended in expiration

❗ **Tips & Tricks**

– The middle of the scapula lies 4 FB below the clavicle and 1 FB lateral to the mamillary line

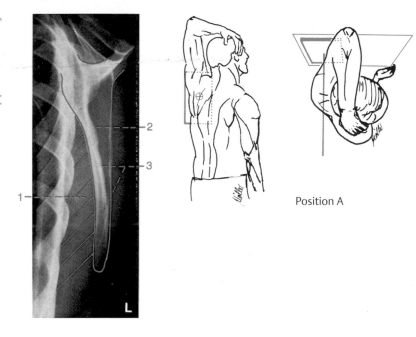

Position A

▶ **Criteria for a Good Radiographic View**

– Clear space between ribs and scapula (1)
– Complete demonstration of the entire scapula (2)
– Lateral and medial border of the scapula superimposed (3)

Position B

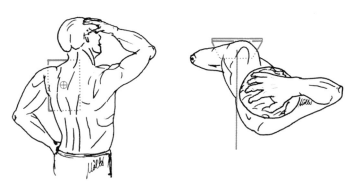

◆ Imaging Technique

Image receiver (e.g., film): size 24 × 30 cm (10 × 12"), portrait
Image receiver dosage (sensitivity class): ≤5 µGy (SC 400)
SID: 115 cm (40")
Bucky: yes (under the table, r 8 [12])
Focal spot size: small (focal spot nominal value ≤1.3)
Exposure: 60–75 kV, automatic, center cell

▨ Patient Preparation

– Remove jewelry (necklace, earrings)
– Remove all clothes from the waist up

▲ Positioning

– Patient with the appropriate shoulder lateral to the upright cassette stand
– Hand on that side placed on top of the head (A) or resting on the hip (B)
  (arm abducted); the other shoulder turned slightly forward (arm of the
  unaffected side held in front), so that medial and lateral borders of the
  scapula to be examined are superimposed (check by palpating between
  thumb and forefinger)
– Lower cassette border 2–4 FB below the inferior angle of the scapula
– Gonads shielded (small lead apron, on the side)

● Alignment

– Projection: tangential to the scapula (slightly oblique lateral, perpendicu-
  lar to the film)
– Central ray directed to the midpoint of the scapula (about middle of the
  axilla) and middle of the film
– Centering, collimation, side identification
– Breathing suspended

Variations

– *Leer–Narché oblique shoulder view,* see p. 98
– *Transscapular shoulder view (Y image),* see p. 99

(Continued on pp. 98, 99)

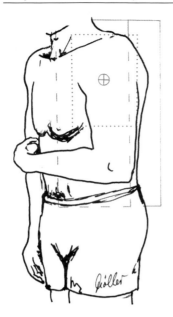

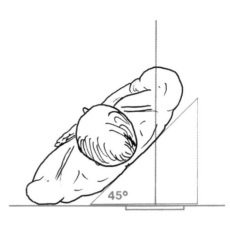

Leer–Narché oblique shoulder view

45°

▲ **Position**

- Patient stands with his or her back on the healthy side obliquely at the vertical Bucky grid (or lies with his or her back on the Bucky table, with the affected side raised)
- The affected side that is being imaged is supported with a 45° wedge cushion (the scapula should be positioned precisely lateral to the film)
- The arm on the affected side hangs down or lies on the abdomen
- Gonads shielded (small lead apron laterally)

● **Alignment**

- Projection: 20° craniocaudad
- Central ray directed vertically through the upper arm to the gap between the ribs and scapula at the center of the film
- Centering, collimation, side identification

Transscapular shoulder view (Y image)

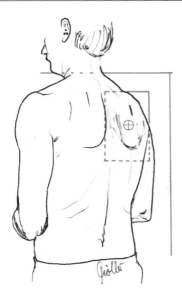

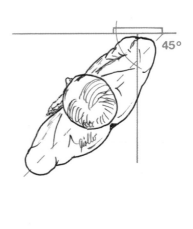

▲ **Position**

- Patient stands with his or her back on the affected side obliquely at the vertical Bucky grid (or lies with his or her back on the Bucky table, with the healthy side raised)
- The healthy side is supported with a 45° wedge cushion (the scapula should be positioned precisely lateral to the film)
- The arm on the affected side hangs down
- Gonads shielded (small lead apron laterally)

● **Alignment**

- Projection: 0° (or 10–15° craniocaudad as a supraspinatus tunnel image)
- Central ray directed vertically through the upper arm to the gap between the ribs and scapula at the center of the film
- Centering, collimation, side identification

▶ **Criteria for a good radiographic view (in both alignments)**

- The scapula, acromion, and coracoid process form a "Y" shape, which is manually projected (no superimposed ribs). The glenoid fossa and the head of the humerus are located at the intersection on the Y.
- Advantages
- The Leer–Narché and Y views are helpful for assessment when there is suspected shoulder dislocation or for a check-up examination after repositioning.

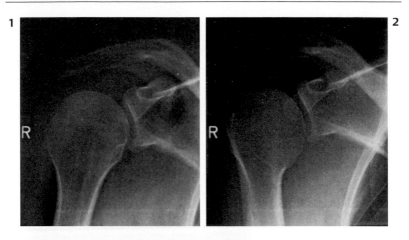

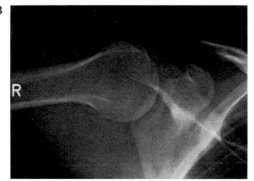

▶ **Criteria for a Good Radiographic View**

– Complete and unobstructed visualization of the head of the humerus and of the shoulder joint

❗ Tips & Tricks

– Center of the humeral head = 3 FB below the clavicle
– Use an intravenous infusion pole for something to hold onto

◆ **Imaging Technique**

Image receiver (e.g., film): size 18×24 cm (8×10"), landscape or 24×30 cm (10×12"), portrait
Image receiver dosage (sensitivity class): ≤5 µGy (SC 400)
SID: 115 cm (40")
Bucky: yes (under the table, r 8 [12])
Focal spot size: small (focal spot nominal value ≤1.3)
Exposure: 60–75 kV, automatic, center cell

▨ **Patient Preparation**

– Remove jewelry (necklace, earrings)
– Remove all clothes from the waist up

▲ **Positioning**

Positions 1 and 2
– Patient stands with the scapula flat against the vertical cassette stand, the opposite side of the back is turned 45° away from the stand
– The arm on the affected side is placed adjacent to the cassette, the elbow is flexed 90°
– Internal rotation (1): forearm is placed on the abdomen
– External rotation (2): forearm is turned out (and may hold on to the cassette stand)
Position 3
– Abduction (3): back flat against the cassette stand (straight, not rotated), arm abducted at a right angle, forearm flexed 90° and extended upward, palm of the hand turned forward (may hold on to an intravenous infusion pole, for instance)
– Upper cassette border 1–2 FB above the superior margin of the shoulder
– Compensating filter for positions 1 and 2
– Gonads shielded (lead apron)

● **Alignment**

– Projection: for 1 and 2: oblique ventrodorsal (AP), 15–20° craniocaudad
– For 3, ventrodorsal, perpendicular to the middle of the cassette
– Central ray for 1 and 2 directed to the center of the head of the humerus and middle of the film; for 3, perpendicular to the joint space
– Centering, collimation, side identification
– Breathing suspended in expiration (Continued on pp. 102, 103)

Projection for positions 1 and 2 (for position 3 = vertical = dotted line)

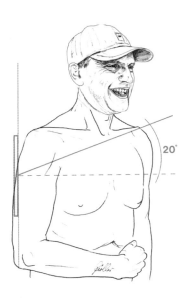

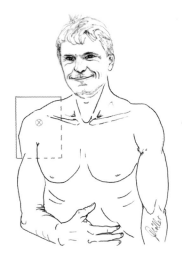

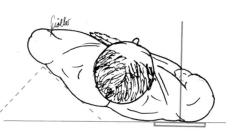

Position 1

Position 2

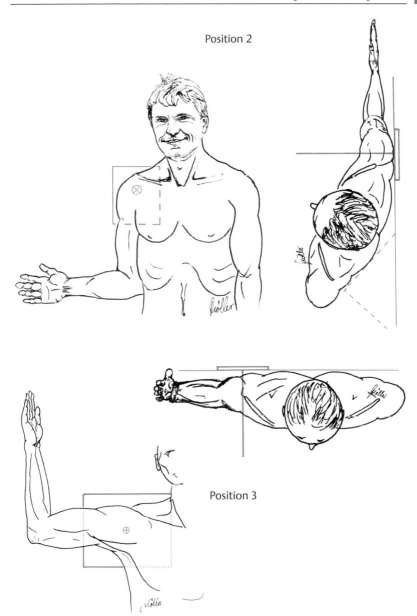

Position 3

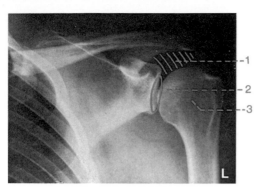

▶ **Criteria for a Good Radiographic View**

– Complete, unobstructed view of the humeral head and shoulder joint (3)
– Glenoid fossa linear or small oval (2)
– Clear view of the subacromial space (1)

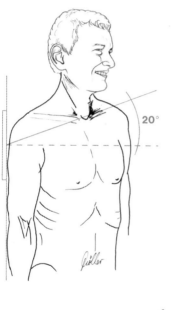

20°

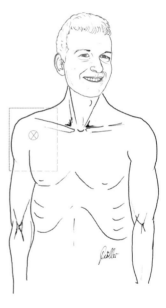

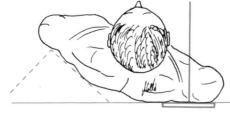

◆ Imaging Technique

Image receiver (e.g., film): size 18 × 24 cm (8 × 10"), portrait
Image receiver dosage (sensitivity class): ≤ 5 µGy (SC 400)
SID: 115 cm (40")
Bucky: yes (under the table, r 8 [12])
Focal spot size: small (focal spot nominal value ≤ 1.3)
Exposure: 60–75 kV, automatic, center cell

■ Patient Preparation

– Remove all clothes from the waist up and all jewelry

▲ Positioning

– Scapula adjacent to and parallel to the cassette, opposite side rotated
  about 45° away from the upright stand (use sponge wedge for support)
– Arm along the side of the body, hanging down, hand supinated
– Head turned the other way (for radiation protection)
– Upper cassette border 1–2 FB above the superior margin of the shoulder
– Shoulder filter, if needed
– Gonads shielded (lead apron)

● Alignment

– Projection: oblique ventrodorsal (AP) (perhaps 20° craniocaudad, although
  not in cases of possible fracture or dislocation)
– Central ray perpendicular to the joint space, and directed to the middle of
  the film
– Centering, collimation, side identification
– Breath held after expiration

Variation

Shoulder in two planes
– Extend the arm straight upward (above the head), otherwise as above
  (shoulder, axial projection, see p. 107)
Glenohumeral joint, profile view, Bernageau position
– Shoulder to be examined turned to the stand
– Arm in maximal abduction, forearm extended above the head, opposite
  side rotated about 20–30° anteriorly
– Projection: lateral, 25–30° craniocaudad
– Central ray 2 cm below the skin fold or the top of the acromion and 2 cm
  towards the spine, directed to the middle of the cassette
Grashey position (lateral process of the scapula)
– Affected arm in internal rotation, projection perpendicular to the film,
  otherwise as above

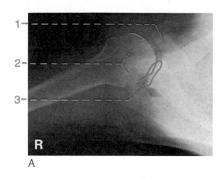

A

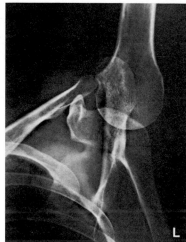

C

▶ **Criteria for a Good Radiographic View**

– Joint surfaces (outlined) and joint space well demonstrated
– Unobstructed view of the coracoid process (1)
– Acromioclavicular joint projected over the humerus (2)
– Inferior glenoid rim clearly demonstrated (3)

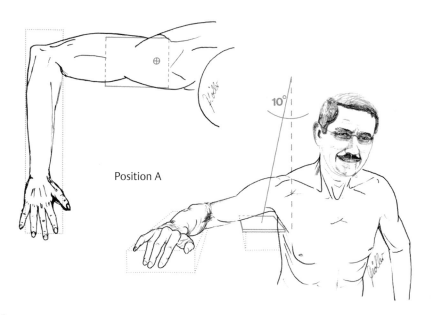

Position A

10°

◆ Imaging Technique

Image receiver (e. g., film): size 18 × 24 cm (8 × 10"), portrait
Image receiver dosage (sensitivity class): ≤ 5 μGy (SC 400)
SID: 105 cm (40")
Bucky: no (tabletop technique)
Focal spot size: small (focal spot nominal value ≤ 1.3)
Exposure: 65–70 kV; __ mAs, __ mAs, __ mAs or (for position C) automatic, center cell

▦ Patient Preparation

– Remove jewelry (necklace, earrings)
– Remove all clothes from the waist up

▲ Positioning

– A. Patient sits at the side of the table; the arm is abducted about 45°, elbow flexed 90°, forearm lies on the table (cassette may be supported), forearm pronated and parallel to the plane of the table
– B. Patient supine, shoulder and upper arm supported, upper arm abducted 90°, forearm supinated (palm of the hand turned up), elevated on wooden board. Cassette placed in vertical position, cephalad, on the radial side of the shoulder, and supported with sandbags. Patient's head inclined all the way to the opposite side
– C. Patient with the back to the stand, arm on the affected side raised vertically, forearm flexed 90° at the elbow and placed on top of the head. Patient's head inclined to the opposite side
– Gonads shielded (lead apron)

● Alignment

– Projection:
  A. Oblique, 5–10°, from cranial–medial to caudal lateral
  B. Oblique, 5–10°, from caudal–lateral to cranial–medial
  C. Vertical ventrodorsal (AP)
– Central ray directed to the center of the joint space and middle of the film
– Centering, collimation, side identification
– Breath held after expiration

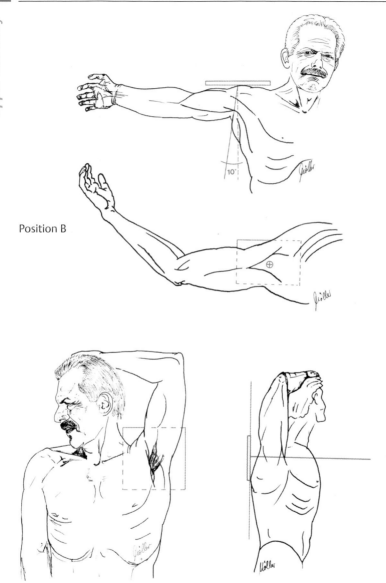

Position B

Position C

◆ Imaging Technique

Image receiver (e.g., film): size 18×24 cm (8×10"), landscape
Image receiver dosage (sensitivity class): ≤5 µGy (SC 400)
SID: 105 cm (40")
Bucky: no (tabletop technique)
Focal spot size: small (focal spot nominal value ≤1.3)
Manual exposure: 50–65 kV; 10 mAs, __ mAs, __ mAs

▨ Patient Preparation

– Remove jewelry (necklace, earrings)
– Remove all clothes from the waist up

▲ Positioning

Hermodsson position
– Supine, hand of the side being examined resting on the opposite shoulder
– Cassette perpendicular to the table behind the shoulder, parallel to the clavicle (lateral side of the cassette moved about 20° toward the head)
Johner position
– Supine, upper arm of the side being examined along the side, forearm flexed 90°, resting on the abdomen
– Cassette on the table behind the shoulder, perpendicular to the central ray
– Have patient turn the head to the other side (radiation protection)
– Gonads shielded (large lead apron)

● Alignment

1 (Hermodsson)
– Projection: parallel to the table, 20° lateromedial
– Central ray perpendicular to the cassette, directed to the midpoint of the humeral head and the middle of the cassette
2 (Johner)
– Projection: oblique horizontal, 20° from lateral to medial, and 20° from caudal to cranial, to the axis of the upper arm of the same side (from laterodorsal to mediocranial)
– Central ray perpendicular to the middle of the cassette
– Centering, collimation, side identification
– Breath held after expiration

(Continued on pp. 110, 111)

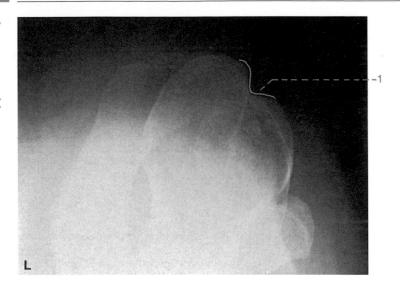

▶ **Criteria for a Good Radiographic View**

– Bicipital groove free of superimposed shadows (1)

Variations

West Point view

– Prone, upper part of the body on broad sponge pad, the arm being examined hanging straight down
– Cassette perpendicular to the table, upright on edge behind the shoulder
– Projection: inferior oblique, 25° from posterior to anterior, and 25° from lateral to medial
– Central ray directed to the joint space and middle of the cassette

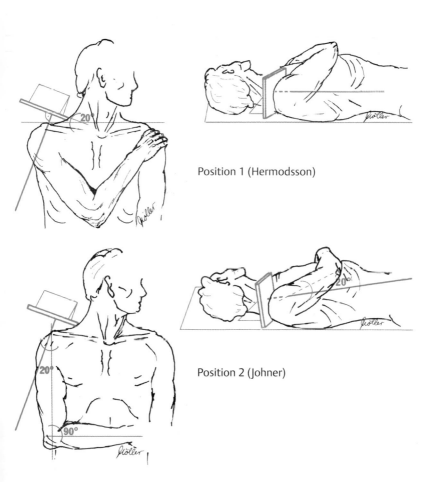

Position 1 (Hermodsson)

Position 2 (Johner)

Upper Extremity

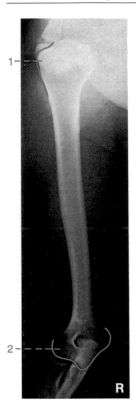

▶ **Criteria for a Good Radiographic View**

- Complete visualization of the entire humerus, including both joints if possible
- AP projection of the trochlea of the humerus (2)
- The greater tubercle presents as the lateral border (1)

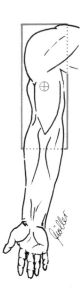

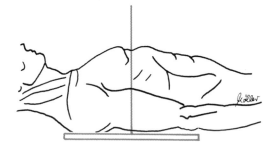

◆ Imaging Technique

Image receiver (e. g., film): size 18×43 cm (7×17") or 20×40 cm (8×16"), portrait

Image receiver dosage (sensitivity class): ≤5 µGy (SC 400), use of compensating screen possible, +/–, plus up

SID: 115 cm (40") or 105 cm (40")

Bucky: yes/no (under the table/tabletop technique)

Focal spot size: small (focal spot nominal value ≤1.3)

Exposure: 60–75 kV, automatic, center cell (or manual: 60–75 kV; 20 mAs, __ mAs, __ mAs)

▦ Patient Preparation

- Remove jewelry (necklace, earrings)
- Remove all clothes from the waist up

▲ Positioning

- Patient with the back to the stand (on the Bucky table)
- Back of the upper arm placed against the cassette (unaffected side slightly rotated forward or elevated)
- Arm somewhat abducted but in contact with the film
- Hand supinated (palm forward = external rotation)
- Upper cassette border 1–2 FB above the superior border of the shoulder
- Head turned to the opposite side
- Gonads shielded (lead apron)

● Alignment

- Projection: ventrodorsal, perpendicular to the film
- Central ray directed to the midpoint of the upper arm and middle of the cassette
- Centering, collimation, side identification
- Breathing suspended

❗ Tips & Tricks

- If external rotation is too painful, turn the entire body with the healthy side forward (or elevate the side) to bring the upper arm adjacent to the film

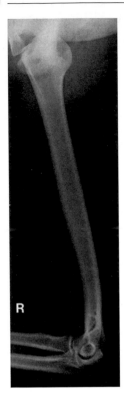

▶ **Criteria for a Good Radiographic View**

– Complete visualization of the entire humerus, including at least one joint (both joints if possible), elbow joint in straight lateral projection

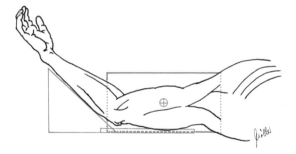

Position A

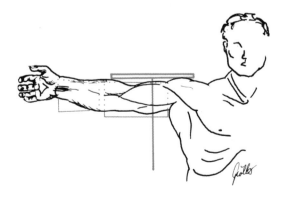

◆ Imaging Technique

Image receiver (e.g., film): size 18 × 43 cm (7 × 17"), portrait
Image receiver dosage (sensitivity class): ≤ 5 µGy (SC 400), use of compensating screen possible, +/−, plus up
SID: 115 cm (40") or 105 cm (40")
Bucky: yes (no)
Focal spot size: small (focal spot nominal value ≤ 1.3)
Exposure: 60–75 kV, automatic, center cell (manual: 66 kV; 20 mAs, __ mAs, __ mAs)

▣ Patient Preparation

- Remove jewelry (necklace, earrings)
- Remove all clothes from the waist up

▲ Positioning

- A. Patient supine, upper arm abducted 90°, forearm supinated (elevated and supported on a wooden board), palm of the hand turned up. Cassette placed on edge against the radial side of the upper arm (from cephalad, so to speak), vertical, and supported with sandbags
- B. Patient sits at the side of the table, upper arm abducted 90°, elbow flexed 90°, forearm rests on the table in the same plane as the upper arm (support if necessary), hand extended straight
- C. Patient with the back to the stand (unaffected side slightly raised), upper arm abducted 90° and rotated externally (forearm elevated, elbow flexed 90°, back of the forearm adjacent to the upright stand)
- Head turned to the opposite side
- Gonads shielded (large lead apron)

● Alignment

- Projection: lateral (at the sagittal level), perpendicular to the film (projection A from the front, B from below, C from above)
- Central ray to midhumerus and middle of the film
- Centering, collimation, side identification
- Breath held after expiration

Position B

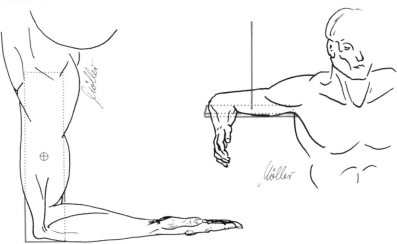

Position C

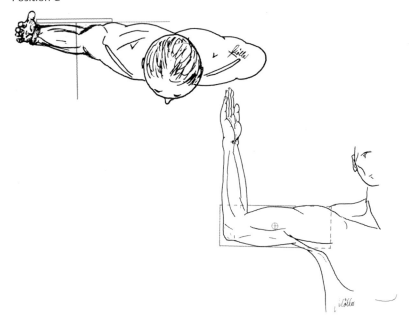

Variation

If the patient is unable to abduct the upper arm:

- Patient supine, upper portion of the body elevated (on a long sponge pad), arm along the side of the body, hand supinated
- Cassette on edge, upright between the chest wall and the inside of the upper arm, pushed as far into the axilla as possible
- Lateral projection, otherwise as above

! Tips & Tricks

- Use intravenous infusion pole for the hand to hold onto
- If there is no compensating screen available, use a bag with rice flour or a wedge filter

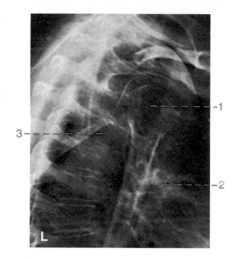

▶ **Criteria for a Good Radiographic View**

- Projection of the humeral head (1) and humerus (2) between the dorsal spine (3) and the sternum (by slightly rotating the unaffected side posteriorly)

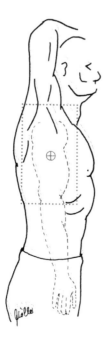
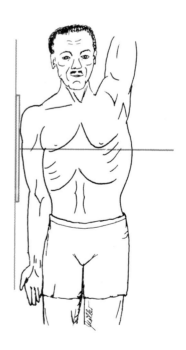

◆ Imaging Technique

Image receiver (e.g., film): size 24×30 cm (10×12"), portrait
Image receiver dosage (sensitivity class): ≤5 µGy (SC 400)
SID: 115 cm (40")
Bucky: yes (under the table)
Focal spot size: large (focal spot nominal value: ≤1.3)
Exposure: 75–85 kV, automatic, center cell

▨ Patient Preparation

– Remove jewelry (necklace, earrings)
– Remove all clothes from the waist up

▲ Positioning

– Patient stands sideways, with the affected shoulder turned to the stand
– Ipsilateral arm hanging down, hand supinated
– Contralateral arm extended above the head
– Unaffected shoulder rotated slightly back
– Upper cassette border 1–2 FB above the superior border of the shoulder
– Gonads shielded (small lead apron)

● Alignment

– Projection: lateral, perpendicular to the film
– Central ray directed to the humeral head being examined (midpoint between the axilla and the nipple of the unaffected side) and middle of the cassette
– Centering, collimation, side identification
– Breathing suspended

❗ Tips & Tricks

– Use the vertigraph for centering by positioning the center photocell over the head of the humerus, then aligning the X-ray tube with the center of the vertigraph

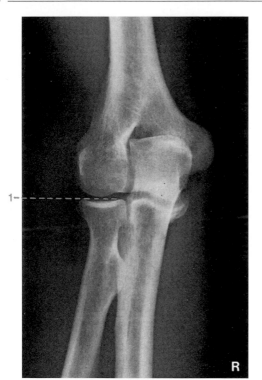

▶ **Criteria for a Good Radiographic View**

– Joint space in the center of the film and clearly demonstrated (1)

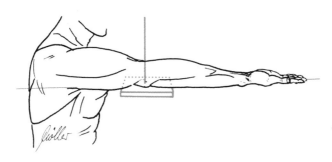

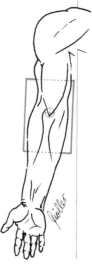

◆ **Imaging Technique**

Image receiver (e.g., film): size 18×24 cm (10×12") or 24×30 cm (10×12"), landscape (divided)
Image receiver dosage (sensitivity class): ≤10 μGy (SC 200)
SID: 105 cm (40")
Bucky: no
Focal spot size: small (focal spot nominal value 0.6 [≤1.3])
Manual exposure: 50–60 kV; 5 mAs; __ mAs, __ mAs

■ **Patient Preparation**

– Remove everything from the arm

▲ **Positioning**

– Patient sits at the side of the table (legs *not* under the table)
– Elbow joint extended, rests with the posterior (dorsal) surface on the cassette, palm turned up (supinated)
– Shoulder, elbow joint, and wrist joint in the same plane, either elevated (sponge or box), or patient's adjustable stool lowered
– Gonads shielded (large lead apron)

● **Alignment**

– Projection: ventro-(volo-)dorsal, perpendicular to the film
– Central ray directed to the middle of the elbow joint and of the cassette
– Centering, collimation, side identification

❗ **Tips & Tricks**

– Put a sandbag on the wrist
– If patient cannot fully extend the elbow, two exposures should be made: one each of the upper arm and of the forearm, each placed on the film

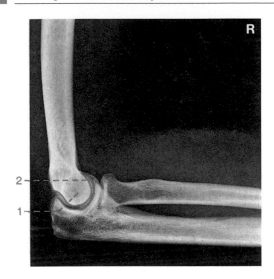

▶ **Criteria for a Good Radiographic View**

- True lateral projection
- Humeroulnar joint space sharply outlined (2)
- Humeral condyles superimposed (1)

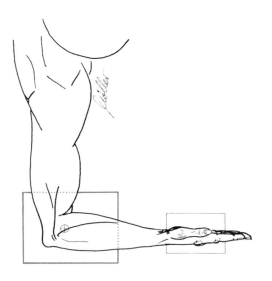

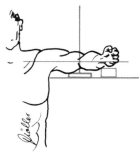

◆ Imaging Technique

Image receiver (e. g., film): size 18×24 cm (8 × 10") or 24×30 cm (10×12"), landscape (divided)
Image receiver dosage (sensitivity class): ≤10 µGy (SC 200)
SID: 105 cm (40")
Bucky: no
Focal spot size: small (focal spot nominal value 0.6 [≤1.3])
Manual exposure: 50–60 kV; 5 mAs; __ mAs, __ mAs

▨ Patient Preparation
- Remove everything from the arm

▲ Positioning
- Patient sits at the side of the table (legs *not* under the table)
- Upper arm and forearm in the same plane (either supported on box or stool lowered)
- Elbow joint flexed 90°, rests with the inside (inferior border) on the cassette
- Wrist in lateral position (thumb up)
- Gonads shielded (large lead apron)

● Alignment
- Projection: lateral radioulnar, perpendicular to film
- Central ray directed to the midpoint of the elbow joint, near the center of the film
- Centering, collimation, side identification

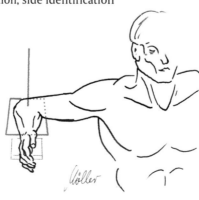

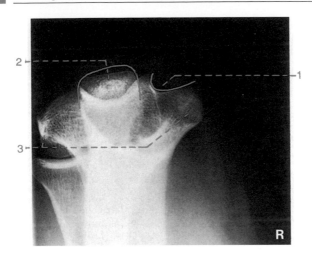

▶ **Criteria for a Good Radiographic View**

- Tangential projection of the ulnar sulcus (1)
- Olecranon (2), trochlea, and the epicondyles (3) are well visualized
- Arm and forearm are superimposed

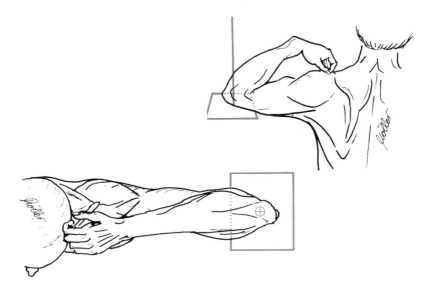

◆ Imaging Technique

Image receiver (e.g., film): size 13×18 cm (8×10") portrait or 18×24 cm (8×10") landscape

Image receiver dosage (sensitivity class): ≤10 µGy (SC 200)

SID: 105 cm (40")

Bucky: no

Focal spot size: small (focal spot nominal value 0.6 [≤1.3])

Manual exposure: 50–60 kV; 5 mAs, __ mAs, __ mAs

▦ Patient Preparation

– Remove everything from the arm

▲ Positioning

– Patient sits at the side of the table
– Arm abducted at a right angle
– Distal portion of the upper arm rests on the cassette
– Elbow joint in maximal flexion (inside of the hand on the shoulder)
– Gonads shielded (large lead apron)

● Alignment

– Projection: perpendicular (ulnohumeral) to the olecranon and to the film
– Central ray directed to the elbow joint (about 2 FB below the olecranon) and to the middle of the film
– Centering, collimation, side identification

Variation

– Patient sits with the back to the table
– Forearm is placed on the cassette, the upper arm is at a 25–30° angle to the vertical plane
– Projection humeroulnar (otherwise as above)

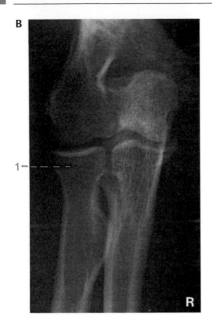

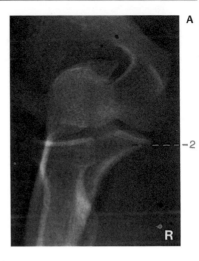

▶ **Criteria for a Good Radiographic View**

– Clear demonstration of the radial head (1) and of the coronoid process of the ulna (2)

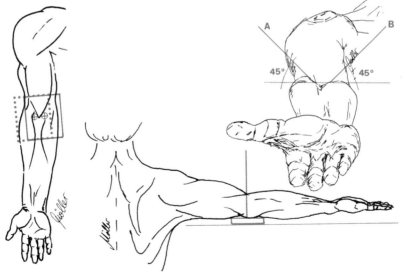

Imaging Technique

Image receiver (e.g., film): size 18×24 cm (8×10"), portrait
Image receiver dosage (sensitivity class): ≤10 µGy (SC 200)
SID: 105 cm (40")
Bucky: no
Focal spot size: small (focal spot nominal value 0.6 [≤1.3])
Manual exposure: 50–60 kV; 5 mAs, __ mAs, __ mAs

Patient Preparation

– Remove everything from the arm

Positioning

– Patient sits at the side of the table (legs *not* under the table)
– The extended elbow joint rests with the posterior (dorsal) surface on the cassette, palm turned up (supinated)
– Shoulder, elbow joint, and wrist joint in the same plane, either elevated (sponge or box) or patient's adjustable stool lowered
– Gonads shielded (large lead apron)

Alignment

Radial head (B)
– Projection: oblique, 45° ulnoradial (medioventral–laterodorsal)
– Central ray directed to the middle of the elbow joint, 1 cm to the ulnar side (toward little finger), and middle of the film
Coronoid process of the ulna (A)
– Projection: oblique, 45° radioulnar (lateroventral–mediodorsal)
– Central ray directed to the middle of the elbow joint, 1 cm to the radial side (toward the thumb)
– Collimate closely to the size of the part and identify the sides

Tips & Tricks

– Midpoint of the elbow joint: transverse centering about 1 FB below the medial epicondyle of the humerus
– Place a sandbag on the wrist

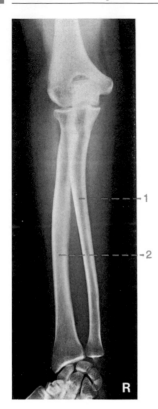

▶ **Criteria for a Good Radiographic View**

– Ulna (1) and radius (2) visualized in their entire length, without being superimposed, and with at least one joint demonstrated (A = with the wrist joint, B = with the elbow joint)

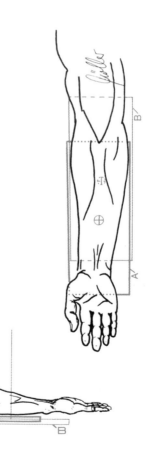

◆ Imaging Technique

Image receiver (e.g., film): size 24×30 cm (10×12"), portrait: (divided; one half covered with a lead mask)
Image receiver dosage (sensitivity class): ≤10 µGy (SC 200)
SID: 105 cm (40")
Bucky: no
Focal spot size: small (focal spot nominal value 0.6 [≤1.3])
Manual exposure: 50–60 kV, 5 mAs, __ mAs, __ mAs

▨ Patient Preparation

- Remove everything from the arm
- Remove jewelry

▲ Positioning

- Patient sits at the side of the table (legs *not* under the table)
- The extended forearm rests with the posterior (dorsal) surface on the cassette
- Palm turned up (supinated)
- Shoulder, elbow joint, and wrist joint in the same plane, either elevated (sponge) or patient's adjustable stool lowered
- Gonads shielded (large lead apron)

● Alignment

- Projection: ventro-(volo-)dorsal, perpendicular to the film
- Central ray directed to the middle of the forearm and of the film
- Centering, collimation, side identification

❗ Tips & Tricks

- Immobilize the fingers with a sandbag
- Use a bag with rice flour to compensate for density differences

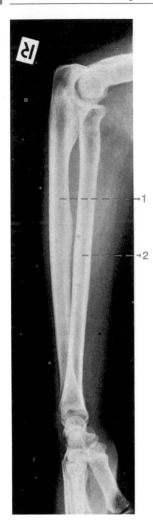

▶ **Criteria for a Good Radiographic View**

- Ulna (1) and radius (2) straight lateral (their distal third superimposed)
- Wrist and elbow joint in straight lateral projection

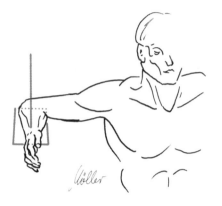

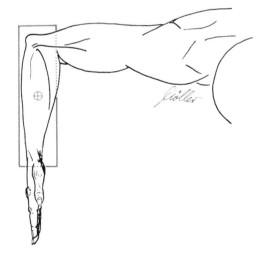

◆ Imaging Technique

Image receiver (e. g., film): size 24 × 30 cm (10 × 12"), portrait (divided; one half covered with a lead mask)
Image receiver dosage (sensitivity class): ≤ 10 µGy (SC 200)
SID: 105 cm (40")
Bucky: no (tabletop technique)
Focal spot size: small (focal spot nominal value 0.6 [≤ 1.3])
Manual exposure: 50–60 kV; 5 mAs, __ mAs, __ mAs

■ Patient Preparation

- Remove everything from the arm
- Remove jewelry

▲ Positioning

- Patient sits at the side of the table (legs *not* under the table)
- Arm elevated and abducted, the elbow flexed 90°
- Forearm rests with the ulnar side on the cassette, straight lateral (wrist joint lateral, little finger down, thumb and fingers extended)
- Midforearm centered over the middle of the film
- Gonads shielded (large lead apron)

● Alignment

- Projection: lateral radioulnar, perpendicular to the film
- Central ray directed to the middle of the forearm and middle of the film
- Centering, collimation, side identification

❗ Tips & Tricks

- Rest the fingers against a right-angled sponge wedge
- Use a bag with rice flour to compensate for density differences

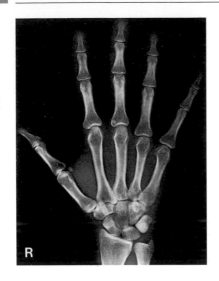

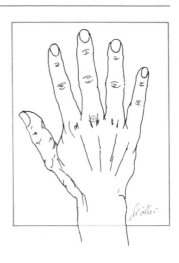

▶ **Criteria for a Good Radiographic View**
- Entire hand visualized, including fingertips and wrist joint

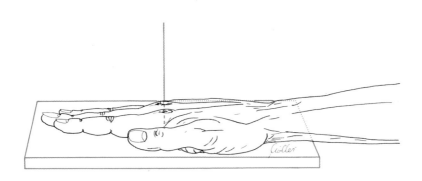

◆ Imaging Technique

Image receiver (e.g., film): size 24×30 cm (10×12"), landscape (divided; one half covered with a lead mask)
Image receiver dosage (sensitivity class): ≤10 μGy (SC 200)
SID: 105 cm (40")
Bucky: no (tabletop exposure)
Focal spot size: small (focal spot nominal value 0.6 [≤1.3])
Manual exposure: 50–60 kV; 3 mAs, __ mAs, __ mAs

▨ Patient Preparation

– Remove everything from the forearm
– Remove jewelry (ring, watch)

▲ Positioning

– Patient sits at the side of the table (legs *not* under the table)
– Forearm rests on the table
– Palm of the hand rests flat on the cassette, fingers slightly spread
– Metacarpophalangeal joint of the middle finger in the center of the film
– Gonads shielded (large lead apron)

● Alignment

– Projection: dorsovolar (PA), perpendicular to the film
– Central ray directed to the metacarpophalangeal joint of the middle finger and middle of the film
– Centering, collimation, side identification

❢ Tips & Tricks

– Place a sandbag across the proximal forearm

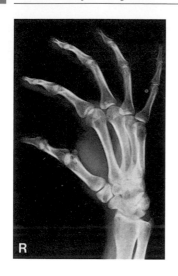

▶ **Criteria for a Good Radiographic View**

- Hand completely visualized, including fingertips and wrist joint

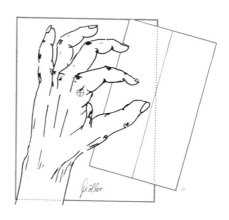

◆ **Imaging Technique**

Image receiver (e.g., film): size 24×30 cm (10×12"), landscape (divided; one half covered with a lead mask)
Image receiver dosage (sensitivity class): ≤10 µGy (SC 200)
SID: 105 cm (40")
Bucky: no
Focal spot size: small (focal spot nominal value 0.6 [≤1.3])
Manual exposure: 50–60 kV; 3 mAs, __ mAs, __ mAs

■ **Patient Preparation**

– Remove everything from the forearm
– Remove jewelry (ring, watch)

▲ **Positioning**

– Patient sits at the side of the table (legs *not* under the table)
– Forearm rests on the table in pronation (palm down)
– Radial aspect of the hand slightly raised (thumb and index finger supported on a sponge wedge)
– Fingers spread and slightly flexed (fanned)
– Metacarpophalangeal joint of the index finger in the center of the film
– Gonads shielded (large lead apron)

● **Alignment**

– Projection: dorsovolar, perpendicular to the film
– Central ray directed to the metacarpophalangeal joint of the index finger in the middle of the film
– Centering, collimation, side identification

Variation

Norgaad position
– Back of the hand rests on the film, thumb side raised about 30° (sponge wedge)
– Fingers slightly bent (ballplayer view)

❗ **Tips & Tricks**

– Place a sandbag across the proximal forearm

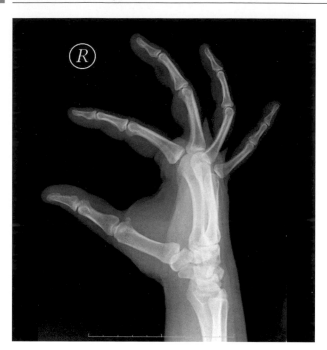

▶ **Criteria for a Good Radiographic View**

– Hand completely visualized, including fingertips and wrist joint
– All of the fingers (except for the thumb) lateral

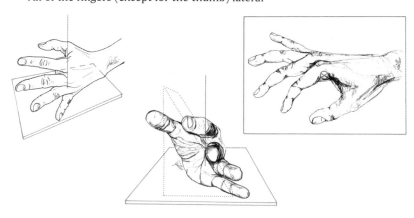

◆ Imaging Technique

Image receiver (e.g., film): size 24×30 cm (10×12"), landscape
Image receiver dosage (sensitivity class): ≤10 µGy (SC 200)
SID: 105 cm (40")
Bucky: no
Focal spot size: small (focal spot nominal value 0.6 [≤1.3])
Manual exposure: 50–60 kV; 10 mAs, __ mAs, __ mAs

▉ Patient Preparation

– Remove everything from the forearm
– Remove jewelry (ring, watch)

▲ Positioning

– Patient sits at the side of the table (legs *not* under the table)
– Ulnar side of forearm rests on the table
– Hand sideways, little finger spread to provide support
– Fingers fanned out (all as lateral as possible, using steeply angled wedge cushion if necessary)
– Metacarpophalangeal joint of the middle finger in the center of the film
– Gonads shielded (large lead apron)

● Alignment

– Projection: lateral (radioulnar), perpendicular to the film
– Central ray directed to the metacarpophalangeal joint of the index finger and middle of the film
– Centering, collimation, side identification

❗ Tips & Tricks

– Support the forearm with a sandbag on the dorsal and volar sides

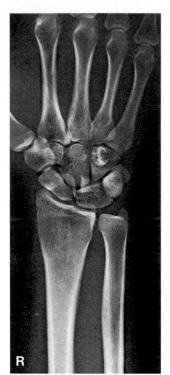

▶ **Criteria for a Good Radiographic View**

– Wrist joint visualized completely (meta-carpals, carpal bones, distal forearm)

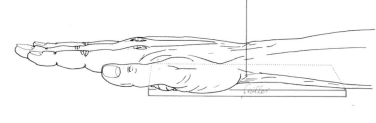

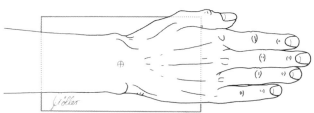

◆ Imaging Technique

Image receiver (e.g., film): size 18 × 24 cm (8 × 10") or 13 × 18 cm (5 × 7"), land-scape (divided; one half covered with lead mask)
Image receiver dosage (sensitivity class): ≤ 10 µGy (SC 200)
SID: 105 cm (40")
Bucky: no
Focal spot size: small (focal spot nominal value 0.6 [≤ 1.3])
Manual exposure: 50–60 kV, 3 mAs, __ mAs, __ mAs

▦ Patient Preparation

– Remove everything from the forearm
– Remove jewelry (ring, watch)

▲ Positioning

– Patient sits at the side of the table (legs *not* under the table)
– Forearm and hand resting on the table in a straight line
– Volar surface of the wrist joint extended and level, resting on the center of the cassette: put a flat sponge pad under the fingers, or have the patient make a flat fist
– Gonads shielded (large lead apron)

● Alignment

– Projection: dorsovolar (PA), perpendicular to the film
– Central ray directed to the center of the wrist joint and middle of the film
– Centering, collimation, side identification

! Tips & Tricks

– Put a sandbag across the proximal forearm
  For taking films through a cast (and in children), use image receiver dos-age (sensitivity class): ≤ 10 µGy (SC 200)

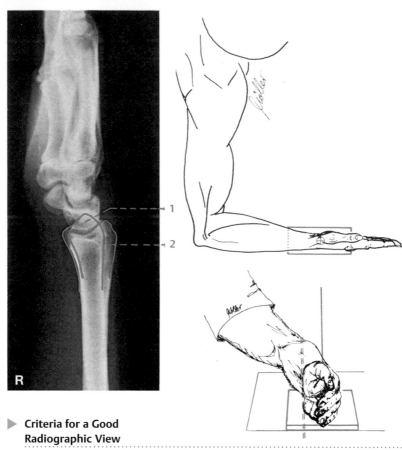

▶ **Criteria for a Good Radiographic View**

– Wrist joint completely visualized, including metacarpals; radius (2) and ulna (1) superimposed

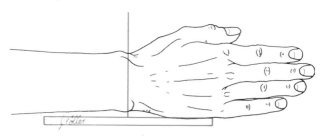

◆ Imaging Technique

Image receiver (e.g., film): size 18×24 cm (8×10"), portrait (divided; one half covered with lead mask)
Image receiver dosage (sensitivity class): ≤10 μGy (SC 200)
SID: 105 cm (40")
Bucky: no (tabletop technique)
Focal spot size: small (focal spot nominal value 0.6 [≤1.3])
Manual exposure: 50–60 kV; 3–4 mAs, __ mAs, __ mAs

■ Patient Preparation

- Remove everything from the forearm
- Remove jewelry (ring, watch)

▲ Positioning

- Patient sits at the side of the table (legs *not* under the table)
- Wrist straight lateral, ulnar (little finger) side rests on the cassette (forearm and hand in one line)
- Thumb on the opposed side, not abducted
- Gonads shielded (large lead apron)

● Alignment

- Projection: lateral (radioulnar), perpendicular to the film
- Central ray directed to the center of the wrist and middle of the film
- Centering, collimation, side identification

▌ Tips & Tricks

- Place a sandbag across the forearm
- Turn the hand so that the thenar eminence (thumb) and hypothenar eminence (little finger) are superimposed
- Patient bends over to the "healthy side" — this facilitates superimposition of the radius and ulna
- Place the hand against a 90° sponge wedge

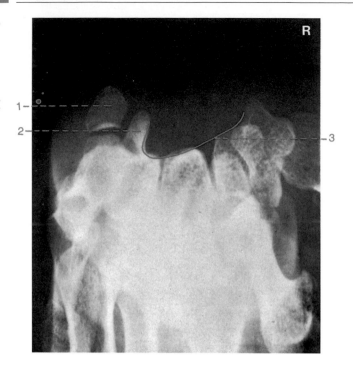

▶ **Criteria for a Good Radiographic View**

– Pisiform bone (1), the hamular process of the hamate (2) and the carpal tunnel (3) are clearly demonstrated

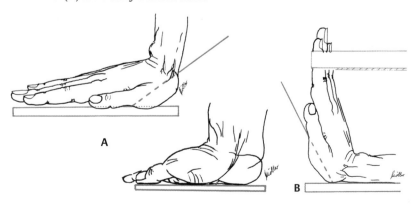

◆ **Imaging Technique**

Image receiver (e.g., film): size 13 × 18 cm (5 × 7") or 18 × 24 cm (8 × 10"), portrait

Image receiver dosage (sensitivity class): ≤ 10 µGy (SC 200)

SID: 105 cm (40")

Bucky: no (tabletop technique)

Focal spot size: small (focal spot nominal value 0.6 [≤ 1.3])

Manual exposure: 50–60 kV; 4–5 mAs, __ mAs, __ mAs

▩ **Patient Preparation**

– Remove everything from the forearm
– Remove jewelry (ring, watch)

▲ **Positioning**

– A. The standing patient puts hand on the cassette in maximal dorsiflexion, palmar surface down
– B. Patient sits at the side of the table (legs *not* under the table)
– Palm of the hand and distal forearm rest on the cassette
– The hand is lifted up and hyperextended in maximal dorsiflexion with the opposite hand (or a band)
– Wrist in the center of the film
– Gonads shielded (large lead apron)

● **Alignment**

– Projection: oblique, 40–45°
– Central ray directed tangentially to the carpal tunnel to the midpoint of the film
– Centering, collimation, side identification

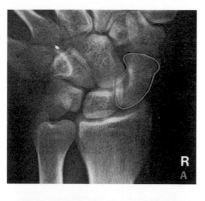

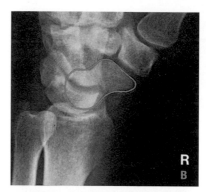

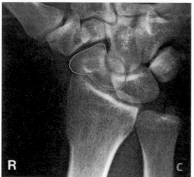

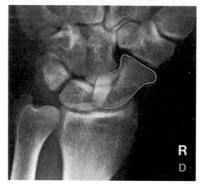

▶ **Criteria for a Good Radiographic View**

– Complete visualization of the navicular bone (outlined) in different projections

– Navicular bone IV (variation): radius and ulna as well as the navicular and lunate are superimposed, the distal portion of the navicular projects along the volar aspect

◆ **Imaging Technique**

Image receiver (e.g., film): size 2 × 13 × 18 cm (2 × 5 × 7"), landscape (divided; one half covered with a lead mask for two projections) or 18 × 24 cm (8 × 10"), landscape (divided for four projections)
Image receiver dosage (sensitivity class): ≤ 10 μGy (SC 200)
SID: 105 cm (40")
Bucky: no (tabletop technique)
Focal spot size: small (focal spot nominal value 0.6 [≤ 1.3])
Manual exposure: 50–60 kV; 3–4 mAs, __ mAs, __ mAs

■ **Patient Preparation**

– Remove everything from the forearm
– Remove jewelry (ring, watch)

▲ **Positioning**

– Patient sits at the side of the table (legs *not* under the table)
– Forearm resting on the table, immobilized with a sandbag
Navicular bone, position I
– Wrist rests with the inferior surface on the middle of the cassette
– Hand in extreme ulnar flexion (thumb and radius form a straight line)
– The metacarpophalangeal joints are extended, interphalangeal joints are flexed
Navicular bone, position II
– Palmar surface of the hand turned down
– Radial side elevated 45° (thumb up), 2nd to the 5th fingers slightly abducted to the ulnar side, supported with a sponge wedge
Navicular bone, position III
– Palmar surface of the hand turned down
– Ulnar side elevated 45° (little finger up), 2nd to the 5th fingers slightly abducted to the ulnar side, supported with a sponge wedge
Navicular bone, position IV
– Palmar surface of the hand rests flat on a 15° sponge wedge
– Fingers slightly abducted to the ulnar side or
Navicular bone, position IV (variation)
– Wrist in true lateral position, ulnar side resting on the middle of the cassette
– Hand hyperextended in dorsiflexion, loose fist
– Gonads shielded (large lead apron)

Navicular bone, position I

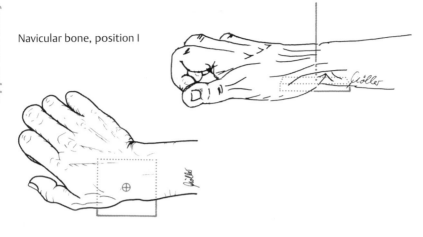

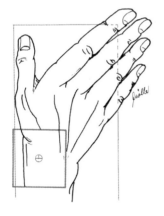

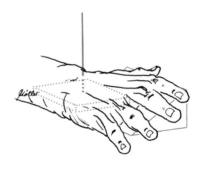

Navicular bone, position II

● **Alignment**

- Projection: dorsovolar, perpendicular to the film
- Central ray directed to the navicular bone (or in variation IV to the center of the wrist and middle of the film)
- Centering, collimation, side identification

! **Tips & Tricks**

- Lateral collimation on the ulnar side not more than to mid-wrist
- Use magnifying technique (e.g., for fractures) (increased object-to-film distance, 0.3 mm smallest focal spot)

Navicular bone, position III

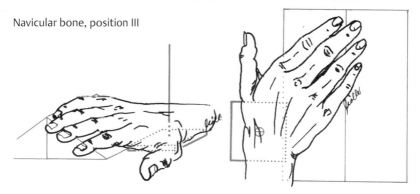

Navicular bone, position IV

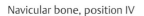
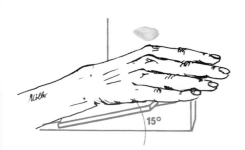
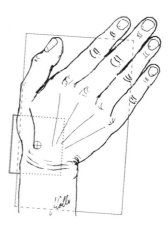

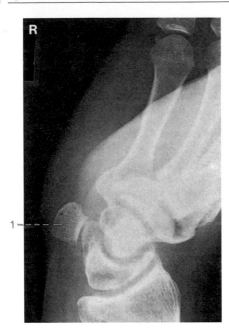

▶ **Criteria for a Good Radiographic View**

– Clear projection of the pisiform bone (1)

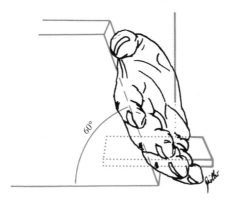

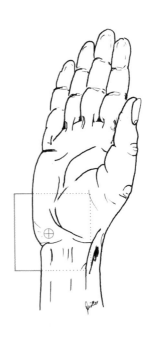

◆ Imaging Technique

Image receiver (e.g., film): size 13 × 18 cm (5 × 7") or 18 × 24 cm (8 × 10"), portrait
Image receiver dosage (sensitivity class): ≤ 10 μGy (SC 200)
SID: 105 cm (40")
Bucky: no (tabletop technique)
Focal spot size: small (focal spot nominal value 0.6 [≤ 1.3])
Manual exposure: 50–60 kV; 3 mAs, __ mAs, __ mAs

▦ Patient Preparation

- Remove everything from the forearm
- Remove jewelry (ring, watch)

▲ Positioning

- Patient sits at the table, placing the dorsum of the hand on the table
- Radial side (thumb up) elevated 60°
- Supported with sponge wedges (e.g., a 15° and a 45° wedge)
- Gonads shielded (large lead apron)

● Alignment

- Projection: oblique radiodorsal, perpendicular to the film
- Central ray directed to the pisiform bone and to the middle of the film
- Centering, collimation, side identification

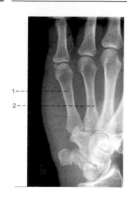

▶ **Criteria for a Good Radiographic View**

- Fifth metacarpal bone completely visualized without superimposition (1), good assessment of the fourth metacarpal (2). Soft-tissue structures well displayed.
- Special aspects of the view: good for assessing injuries to the fourth and fifth metacarpals or for check-up examinations afterward

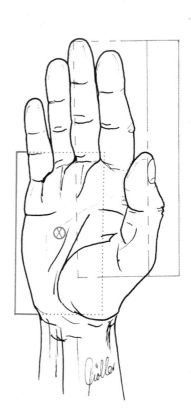

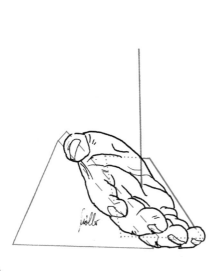

◆ **Imaging Technique**

Image receiver (e.g., film): size 24 × 30 cm (10 × 12"), portrait
Image receiver dosage (sensitivity class): ≤ 10 µGy (SC 200)
SID: 105 cm (41.3")
Bucky: no
Focal spot size: small (focal spot nominal value 0.6 [≤ 1.3])
Manual exposure: 50–60 kV; 10 mAs, __ mAs, __ mAs

■ **Patient Preparation**

– Remove everything from the forearm
– Remove jewelry (ring, watch)

▲ **Positioning**

– Patient sits at the side of the table (legs *not* under the table)
– Ulnar side of forearm (small finger side) rests on the table
– Hand in oblique lateral position, back of the hand supported with a 45°
  wedge cushion
– Support the thumb
– Gonads shielded (large lead apron)

● **Alignment**

– Projection: oblique (palmodorsal), perpendicular to the film
– Central ray directed to the fifth metacarpal bone and middle of the film
– Centering, collimation, side identification (mirror image)

❗ **Tips & Tricks**

– Support the forearm with a sandbag on the dorsal and volar sides

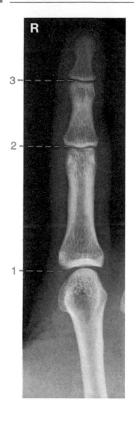

▶ **Criteria for a Good Radiographic View**

– Metacarpophalangeal (1), proximal (2), and distal (3) interphalangeal joints with no superimposition

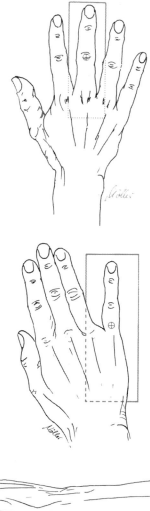

◆ Imaging Technique

Image receiver (e.g., film): size 13 × 18 cm (5 × 7"), portrait (divided; one half covered with lead mask)
Image receiver dosage (sensitivity class): ≤ 10 μGy (SC 200)
SID: 105 cm (40")
Bucky: no (tabletop technique)
Focal spot size: small (focal spot nominal value 0.6 [≤ 1.3])
Manual exposure: 50–60 kV; 1 mAs, __ mAs, __ mAs

▮ Patient Preparation

- Remove everything from the forearm
- Remove jewelry (ring, watch)

▲ Positioning

- Patient sits at the side of the table
- Hand rests with the palmar surface on the cassette
- Finger being examined centered to the midline of the (unmasked half) of the cassette
- The other fingers abducted
- Gonads shielded (lead apron)

● Alignment

- Projection: dorsovolar, perpendicular to the film
- Central ray directed to the proximal interphalangeal (or to the metacarpophalangeal joint, the part of the finger in question = central ray) and to the middle of the cassette
- Sandbag placed over the forearm
- Centering, collimation, side identification

❗ Tips & Tricks

- If the volar side of the finger is injured, place the dorsal side on the film, or use some gauze padding

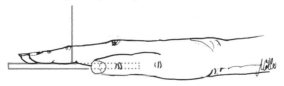

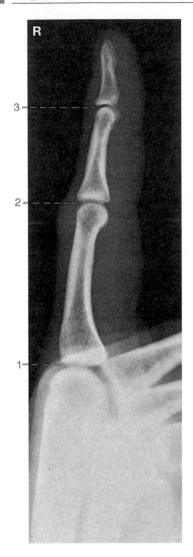

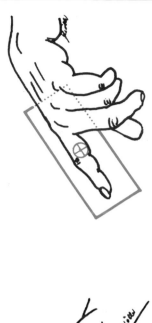

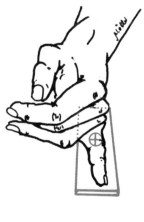

▶ **Criteria for a Good Radiographic View**

– Metacarpophalangeal (1), proximal (2), and distal (3) interphalangeal joints with no superimposition and in true lateral projection

◆ **Imaging Technique**

Image receiver (e.g., film): size 13 × 18 cm (5 × 7"), portrait (divided; one-half covered with lead mask)
Image receiver dosage (sensitivity class): ≤ 10 µGy (SC 200)
SID: 105 cm (40")
Bucky: no (tabletop technique)
Focal spot size: small (focal spot nominal value 0.6 [≤ 1.3])
Manual exposure: 50–60 kV; 1 mAs, __ mAs, __ mAs

▨ **Patient Preparation**

– Remove everything from the forearm
– Remove jewelry (ring, watch)

▲ **Positioning**

– Patient sits at the side of the table (legs *not* under the table)
– Second and 3rd fingers rest on the cassette with their radial side, 4th and 5th fingers with their ulnar side (fingernails straight lateral, 3rd and 4th fingers supported so that the long axis of the entire finger is parallel to the film)
– Adjacent fingers flexed (use bands if necessary)
– Gonads shielded (large lead apron)

● **Alignment**

– Projection: lateral (2nd and 3rd fingers ulnoradial, 4th and 5th fingers radioulnar), perpendicular to the film
– Central ray to the proximal interphalangeal joint and middle of the cassette
– Centering, collimation, side identification

❗ **Tips & Tricks**

– Immobilize the extended finger with a tongue depressor or hold with the fingers of the other hand

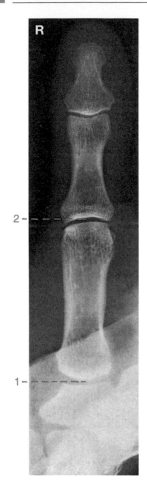

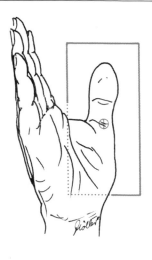

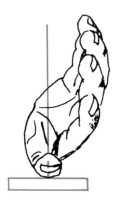

▶ **Criteria for a Good Radiographic View**
....
– Carpometacarpal joint (1) and thumb from the metacarpophalangeal joint (2) to the tip with no superimposition

◆ Imaging Technique

Image receiver (e. g., film): size 13 × 18 cm (5 × 7"), landscape (divided; one half covered with a lead mask)

Image receiver dosage (sensitivity class): ≤ 10 µGy (SC 200)

SID: 105 cm (40")

Bucky: no

Focal spot size: small (focal spot nominal value 0.6 [≤ 1.3])

Manual exposure: 50–60 kV, 1 mAs, __ mAs, __ mAs

■ Patient Preparation

- Remove everything from the forearm
- Remove jewelry (ring, watch)

▲ Positioning

- Patient sits at the side of the table (legs *not* under the table)
- Forearm in maximal internal rotation
- Dorsum of the thumb and metacarpal are resting directly on the cassette
- Maximal pronation, dorsum of the hand supported on a sponge wedge
- Gonads shielded (large lead apron)

● Alignment

- Projection: volodorsal, perpendicular to the film
- Central ray directed to the metacarpophalangeal joint of the thumb and the middle of the cassette
- Centering, collimation, side identification

❗ Tips & Tricks

- The film can also be taken at the upright Bucky stand (cassette centered on the affected part, the arm adducted and flexed, hand rotated inward, dorsum of the thumb placed on the cassette and immobilized)
- If internal rotation is not possible: patient places the hand in a lateral position with the little finger (ulnar) side down, thumb is abducted and placed on the (elevated and supported) cassette
- Sometimes positioning may be more comfortable for the patient if the arm is abducted dorsally (which means that the patient sits with the back to the table; shielding of the gonads must be ensured)

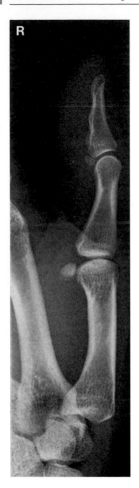

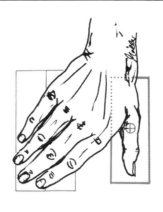

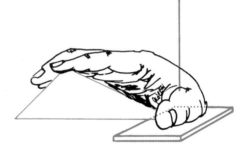

▶ **Criteria for a Good Radiographic View**

– Thumb in true lateral projection, from the carpometacarpal joint to the tip with no superimposition

◆ Imaging Technique

Image receiver (e.g., film): size 13 × 18 cm (5 × 7"), landscape (divided; one half covered with lead mask)
Image receiver dosage (sensitivity class): ≤ 10 µGy (SC 200)
SID: 105 cm (40")
Bucky: no
Focal spot size: small (focal spot nominal value 0.6 [≤ 1.3])
Manual exposure: 50–60 kV; 1 mAs, __ mAs, __ mAs

■ Patient Preparation

– Remove everything from the forearm
– Remove jewelry (ring, watch)

▲ Positioning

– Patient sits at the side of the table (legs *not* under the table)
– The abducted thumb rests with the radial side on the cassette (fingernail straight lateral)
– The other four fingers are elevated and supported on a sponge wedge
– Gonads shielded (large lead apron)

● Alignment

– Projection: lateral (ulnoradial), perpendicular to the film
– Central ray directed to the metacarpophalangeal joint of the thumb and middle of the cassette
– Centering, collimation, side identification

Variations

– With a loosely closed fist (hand arched) and the thumb abducted, the thumb is in a lateral position that requires no sponge support
– Oblique view of the thumb: when the hand lies flat, the thumb is in an oblique position, alignment otherwise as above

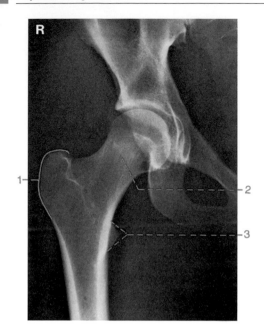

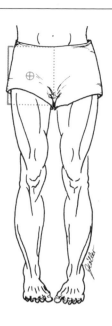

▶ **Criteria for a Good Radiographic View**

– Complete visualization of the hip joint (from the lower portion of the iliac wing to the proximal femur)
– Hip joint in the upper third of the film
– Greater trochanter (1) forms the lateral margin (should not be superimposed on the femoral neck)
– Femoral neck not foreshortened (2)
– Lesser trochanter forms the inner margin (3)

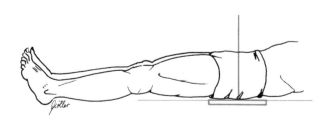

◆ **Imaging Technique**

Image receiver (e.g., film): size 24×30 cm (10×12"), portrait
Image receiver dosage (sensitivity class): ≤5 µGy (SC 400)
SID: 115 cm (40")
Bucky: yes (under the table, r 8 [12])
Focal spot size: large (focal spot nominal value: ≤1.3)
Exposure: 70–80 kV, automatic, center cell

■ **Patient Preparation**

– Remove clothes from the waist down, except underwear

▲ **Positioning**

– Supine, legs straight (parallel to the longitudinal axis of the body)
– Feet turned inward (large toes touching) (no internal rotation if a fracture is suspected)
– Gonads shielded

● **Alignment**

– Projection: AP, perpendicular to the film
– Central ray to the center of the femoral neck (midinguinal) and the middle of the cassette
– Upper border of the cassette: anterior superior iliac spine
– Centering, collimation, side identification (inferior, lateral)
– Breath held after expiration

Variation

If there is a prosthetic device present
– Use a larger film size (20×40 cm [8×16"])
– Don't use photocell

❚ **Tips & Tricks**

– The femoral artery pulse can be used as a centering aid; it is located over the femoral head
– Put a sandbag across the lower leg

Lower Extremity

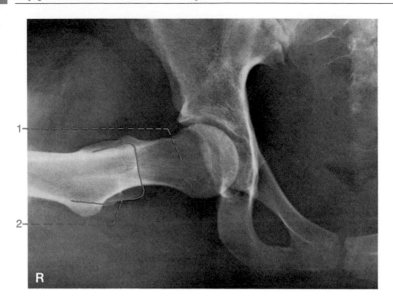

▶ **Criteria for a Good Radiographic View**
- Complete visualization of the hip joint
- Femoral neck and shaft in straight alignment (1)
- The greater trochanter (2) is partly projected behind the femoral neck

◆ Imaging Technique

Image receiver (e.g., film): size 24×30 cm (10×12"), portrait
Image receiver dosage (sensitivity class): ≤5 µGy (SC 400)
SID: 115 cm (40")
Bucky: yes (under the table, r 8 [12])
Focal spot size: large (focal spot nominal value: ≤1.3)
Exposure: 70–80 kV, automatic, center cell

▦ Patient Preparation

- Remove clothes from the waist down, except underwear

▲ Positioning

- Supine position
- The affected hip joint in 45° flexion and 45° abduction
- Thigh supported on padding
- Gonads shielded (lead apron, testicle cups)

● Alignment

- Projection: AP, perpendicular to the film
- Central ray directed to the center of the femoral neck (midinguinal) and the middle of the cassette (anterior superior iliac spine at the upper border of the cassette)
- Centering, collimation, side identification
- Breath held after expiration

Variations

Lauenstein I
- Supine position, hip and knee flexed 45°
- Opposite side elevated until the affected hip is in a lateral position

Lauenstein II
- Supine position, hip and knee flexed so that the sole of the foot stands on the table
- Leg slightly abducted (bent outward), not rotated externally
- Central ray 2 FB lateral to and above the inguinal midpoint

(Continued on p. 164)

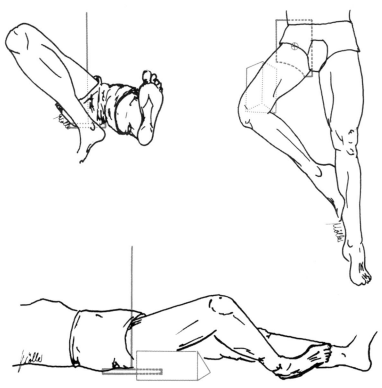

Hip joint, axial, Lauenstein projection

! Tips & Tricks

- If the patient's ability to move is limited, elevate and support the unaffected side
- Put the cassette diagonally into the table tray (angle the tube accordingly) = better positioning, shows more of the femur (the femur projects into the lower lateral corner of the cassette)
- If a prosthetic device is present, a larger cassette (e.g., 18 × 43 cm [7 × 17"]) may be required

◆ Imaging Technique

Image receiver (e.g., film): size 24×30 cm (10×12"), portrait
Image receiver dosage (sensitivity class): ≤5 µGy (SC 400)
SID: 115 cm (40")
Bucky: yes (under the table, r 8 [12])
Focal spot size: large (focal spot nominal value: ≤1.3)
Exposure: 70–80 kV, automatic, center cell

▨ Patient Preparation

- Remove clothes from the waist down, except underwear

▲ Positioning

- Supine position
- 1. Hip joint to be examined flexed 45° (30–60°), foot stands on the table
- 2. Hip joint to be examined extended, foot in slight internal rotation
- Upper border of the cassette at the level of the anterior superior iliac spine
- Gonads shielded (lead apron, testicle cup)

● Alignment

- Projection:
    1. AP, perpendicular to the film
    2. 30° craniocaudad angulation
- Central ray directed to the center of the femoral neck (midinguinal) and middle of the cassette
- Centering, collimation, side identification

Variations

Faux-profile view
- Patient stands sideways with the affected hip turned towards the vertical Bucky stand
- Foot on the affected side parallel to the stand
- The pelvic half away from the film is rotated back at a 65° angle toward the stand (the healthy leg included)
- Arms above the head
- Central ray directed perpendicularly to the hip to be examined (about 2 FB medial to the inguinal midpoint)

(Continued on pp. 166, 167)

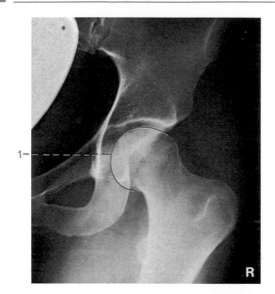

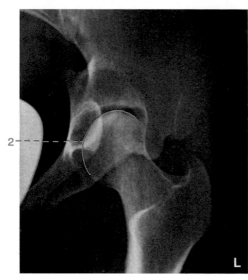

▶ **Criteria for a Good Radiographic View**

- Joint space in the center of the film
- Contour of the femoral head outlined
  (1 = anterior,
   2 = posterior contour)

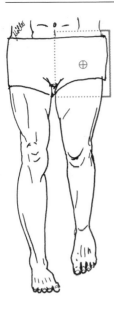

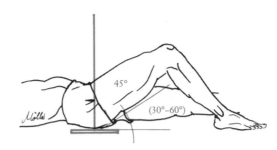

1. Contour view of the femoral head
   (anterior contour)

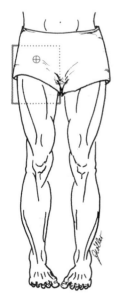

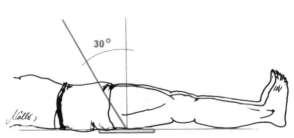

2. Contour view of the femoral head
   (posterior contour)

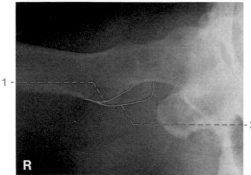

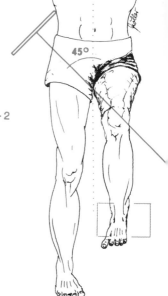

▶ **Criteria for a Good Radiographic View**

– Complete visualization of the hip joint
– Femoral neck in the center of the film, un-foreshortened and without superimposition
– Trochanters projected "underneath" (1 and 2)

● **Alignment**

– Projection: oblique, about 45°, from caudo-medial to craniolateral, perpendicular to the film
– Central ray directed to the center of the femoral neck (midinguinal)
– Centering, collimation, side identification

! **Tips & Tricks**

– Cassette must be placed well inside the waist
– Buttocks supported so that the femoral neck is centered over the midpoint of the film
– If no screen is being used, place bags with rice flour on the inside of the thigh to compensate for differences in density

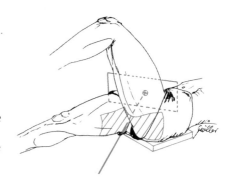

Lower Extremity

◆ **Imaging Technique**

Image receiver (e.g., film): size 24×30 cm (10×12"), portrait
Image receiver dosage (sensitivity class): ≤5 µGy (SC 400); if compensating screen is used, +/–, plus up
SID: 105 cm (40")
Bucky: grid cassette, tabletop technique
Focal spot size: large (focal spot nominal value: ≤1.3)
Manual exposure: 85 kV; 30 mAs, __ mAs, __ mAs

▨ **Patient Preparation**

– Remove clothes from the waist down, except underwear

▲ **Positioning**

– Supine position, buttocks supported (elevated)
– Hip joint to be examined is extended, rotated medially by perhaps 10° (not when a fracture is present)
– The healthy leg is completely flexed at the hip (and knee joint) and elevated (for instance, on a wooden box)
– The cassette is placed upright against the outside of the affected hip, perpendicular to the plane of the table and parallel to the femoral neck (at an angle of about 45° toward the longitudinal axis), and is supported in the vertical position with a sandbag or wedge pillow

Variations

Hips in sitting position, semiaxial projection

– Patient seated with the back to the vertical Bucky stand (on a wooden box, for instance), pelvis adjacent to the cassette tray. Both thighs abducted exactly 20° each from the median sagittal plane
– Image receiver (e.g., film): size 20×40 cm (8×16") or 18×43 cm (7×17")
– Film speed: 400
– Bucky: yes (upright Bucky stand)
– Exposure: 80 kV, automatic, center cell (lower cassette border 1–2 cm below the seat level)

Antetorsion view of the hips, Rippstein position

– Patient in supine position, leg-holder device brought up to the pelvis
– Legs placed on the holder in such a way that hip and knee are flexed at right angles and both hips are abducted 20° each from the median sagittal plane
– Otherwise same as the sitting view

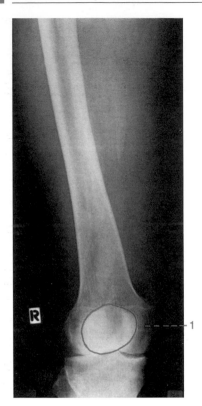

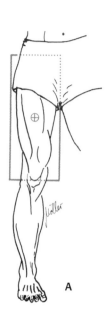

A

▶ **Criteria for a Good Radiographic View**

– Femur exactly AP
– Hip joint (greater trochanter forms the lateral border) or knee joint (patella [1] overlying the middle of the femur) are included in the view

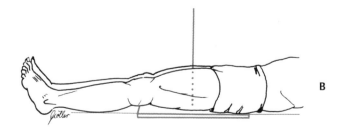

B

◆ Imaging Technique

Image receiver (e.g., film): size 20×40 cm (8×16") or 18×43 cm (7×17"), portrait

Image receiver dosage (sensitivity class): ≤5 μGy (SC 400); if compensating screen is used, +/−, plus up

SID: 115 cm (40")

Bucky: yes (under the table, r 8 [12])

Focal spot size: large (focal spot nominal value: ≤1.3)

Exposure: 70–80 kV, automatic, center cell

■ Patient Preparation

– Remove clothes from the waist down, except underwear

▲ Positioning

– Supine position
– Legs straight, slightly rotated medially
– Contralateral leg somewhat abducted
  Either:
A. *(with hip joint)*
– Upper cassette border at the anterior superior iliac spine; or
B. *(with knee joint)*
– Lower cassette border about 5 cm below the joint space of the knee
– Gonads shielded (lead apron)

● Alignment

– Projection: AP, perpendicular to the film
– Central ray directed to the middle of the cassette
– Centering, collimation, side identification
– Breath held after expiration

Variation

Femur, with both joints
– Image receiver (e.g., film): size 20×60 cm (8×24")
– Upper border: anterior superior iliac spine

❗ Tips & Tricks

– Use either a wedge filter or rice flour to compensate for density differences
– Adjustment of the longitudinal axis of the leg is best done from the foot
– Maintain and immobilize the rotation by placing a sandbag across the lower leg

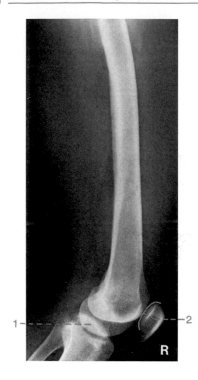

▶ **Criteria for a Good Radiographic View**

– Femur straight lateral
– Hip or knee joint (1) included on the film
– Patella clearly shown (2) (on film that includes the knee joint)

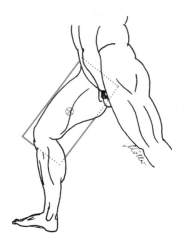

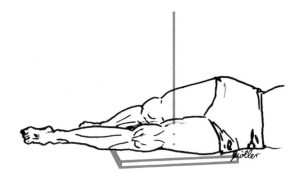

Lower Extremity

◆ Imaging Technique

Image receiver (e. g., film): size 18×43 cm (7×17") or 20×40 cm (8×16"), portrait

Image receiver dosage (sensitivity class): ≤5 µGy (SC 400); if compensating screen is used, +/–, plus up

SID: 115 cm (40")

Bucky: yes (under the table, r 8 [12])

Focal spot size: large (focal spot nominal value: ≤1.3)

Exposure: 70–80 kV for the hip; 60–65 kV for the knee joint, automatic, center cell

▮ Patient Preparation

– Remove clothes from the waist down, except underwear

▲ Positioning

– Patient lies on the side, the leg to be examined is placed in lateral position on the table, hip and knee flexed
– The other leg either:
  A. (Femur, including hip joint) hyperextended and placed behind the leg to be examined (upper cassette border [+] at the level of the anterior superior iliac spine) or
  B. (Femur, including knee joint) strongly flexed, supported, placed in front of the leg to be examined (lower cassette border [–] about 5 cm below the joint space of the knee)
– Gonads shielded (testicle cups for men)

● Alignment

– Projection: mediolateral, perpendicular to the film
– Central ray directed to the middle of the cassette (which is centered in A over the proximal, in B over the distal third of the femur)
– Centering, collimation, side identification
– Breath held after expiration

Variation

– View of the femur with both joints:
– Image receiver (e. g., film): size 20×60 cm (8×24")
– Upper cassette border at the level of the anterior superior iliac spine, otherwise as in A

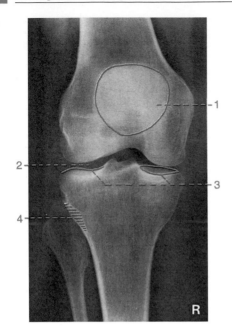

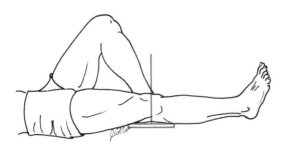

▶ **Criteria for a Good Radiographic View**

- Patella in midline (1)
- Joint space clearly defined (2)
- Planar projection of the tibial plateau
- Tibia superimposed on the medial aspect of the fibular head only

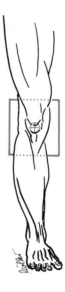

◆ Imaging Technique

Image receiver (e. g., film): size 18×24 cm (8×10"), portrait (or 24×30 cm [10×12"], landscape, divided for two views)
Image receiver dosage (sensitivity class): ≤5 µGy (SC 400)
SID: 115 cm (40") or 105 cm (40")
Bucky: yes (no)
Focal spot size: small (focal spot nominal value: ≤1.3)
Exposure:
- Bucky tray under the table: 60–75 kV, automatic, center cell
  Tabletop technique without Bucky: 50–55 kV; 4–5 mAs, __ mAs, __ mAs

▦ Patient Preparation

- Remove clothes from the waist down, except underwear

▲ Positioning

- Supine position, leg extended, in slight internal rotation (until patella is in midline)
- Other leg abducted
- Lower leg immobilized with sandbag
- Gonads shielded (large lead apron)

● Alignment

- Projection: AP, perpendicular to the film
- Central ray directed to the midpoint of the joint space (2 cm = 1 FB below the superior pole of the patella) and middle of the cassette
- Centering, collimation, side identification

▮ Tips & Tricks

- If the knee cannot be fully extended, support the knee, then move the central ray distally about 1 or 2 cm
- Increase the focal film distance to lessen magnification (exposure correction for manual setting: 1 exposure point for every 10 cm)
- If cruciate ligament injury is suspected, have the patient slightly bend the knee to demonstrate the intercondylar tubercles

Lower Extremity

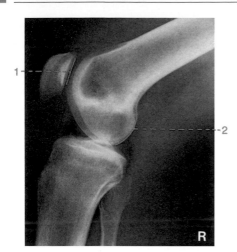

▶ **Criteria for a Good Radiographic View**

– Posterior surface of the patella clearly delineated (1)
– Femoral condyles superimposed (especially dorsal aspect, 2)
– Joint space of the knee clearly visualized
– Tibial tuberosity can be evaluated

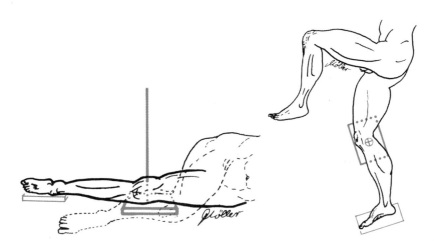

◆ Imaging Technique

Image receiver (e.g., film): size 18×24 cm (8 × 10"), portrait (or 24×30 cm [10 × 12"], landscape; divided for two views)
Image receiver dosage (sensitivity class): ≤5 µGy (SC 400)
SID: 115 cm (40") or 105 cm (40")
Bucky: yes (no)
Focal spot size: small (focal spot nominal value: ≤1.3)
Exposure:
- Bucky tray under the table: 60–75 kV, automatic, center cell
- Tabletop technique without Bucky: 55–70 kV; 4–5 mAs, __ mAs, __ mAs

▨ Patient Preparation

- Remove clothes from the waist down, except underwear

▲ Positioning

- Patient lies on side, the lateral side of the knee is placed on the cassette (or on the table)
- Knee flexed 30° to 45°
- Lower leg parallel to the surface plane (heel/calcaneus supported with a sponge)
- Opposite leg placed in front of the leg to be examined
- Gonads shielded (large lead apron)

● Alignment

- Projection: lateral, perpendicular to the film
- Central ray directed to the midpoint of the joint space (2 cm below the superior pole of the patella) and middle of the cassette
- Centering, collimation, side identification

Variation

- If mobility is restricted, place the cassette upright on its edge and take the film in horizontal projection.

▮ Tips & Tricks

- If there is osteoporosis, reduce the kilovoltage (to about 55 kV)
- Films should not be made too dark, or soft-tissue changes may be missed

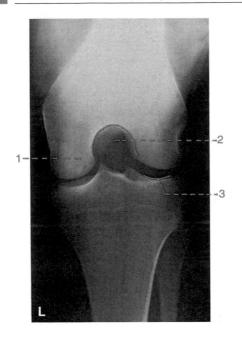

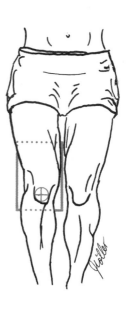

▶ **Criteria for a Good Radiographic View**

- Joint space (intercondylar fossa) clearly defined (2)
- Femoral condyles with no superimposition (1)
- Linear projection of the lateral tibial plateau (3)

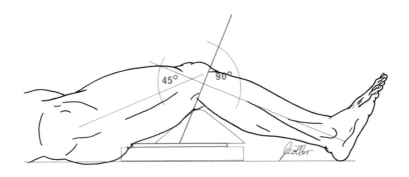

Lower Extremity

◆ **Imaging Technique**

Image receiver (e. g., film): size 18 × 24 cm (8 × 10"), portrait (curved cassette)
Image receiver dosage (sensitivity class): ≤ 5 µGy (SC 400)
SID: 105 cm (40")
Bucky: no (tabletop technique)
Focal spot size: small (focal spot nominal value: ≤ 1.3)
Manual exposure: 50–60 kV; 4 mAs, __ mAs, __ mAs

■ **Patient Preparation**

– Remove clothes from the waist down, except underwear

▲ **Positioning**

– Supine position
Either A:
– Cassette is placed on a sponge pad and under a triangular sponge wedge
– The affected knee is put on the wedge and flexed 45°
– Patella in midline position (leg in slight internal rotation)
– The other leg is abducted
Or B:
– The curved cassette is put over the triangular wedge in the popliteal fossa
– Gonads shielded (large lead apron)

● **Alignment**

– Projection: perpendicular to the axis of the lower leg (about 30–45° caudocephalad toward the film)
– Central ray directed to the midpoint of the joint space (2–3 cm below the
  lower pole of the patella) and the middle of the cassette
– Centering, collimation, side identification

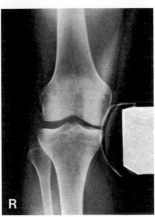

R

▶ **Criteria for a Good Radiographic View**

AP view of the knee:
- Joint space freely visible
- Planar projection of the tibial plateau
- Tibia superimposed only on the medial aspect of the head of the fibula

Lateral view of the knee:
- Posterior surface of the patella clearly delineated
- Femoral condyles largely superimposed
- Joint space of the knee freely visible

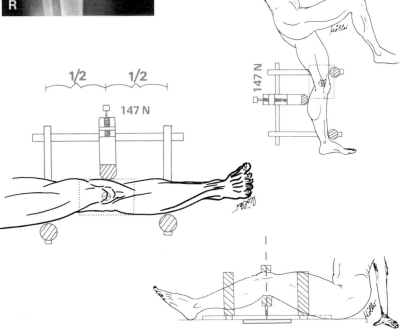

● **Alignment**

- Projection: AP or lateral, perpendicular to the film
- Central ray directed to the midpoint of the joint space (2 cm = 1 FB below the superior pole of the patella and the middle of the cassette)
- Centering, collimation, side identification, notation of the applied pressure (147 N [15 kp])

◆ Imaging Technique

Image receiver (e.g., film): size 18×24 cm (8×10"), portrait (or 24×30 cm [10×12"], landscape, divided for two views)
Image receiver dosage (sensitivity class): ≤5 µGy (SC 400)
SID: 115 cm (40") or 105 cm (40")
Bucky: yes (no)
Focal spot size: small (focal spot nominal value: ≤1.3)
Exposure:
- With Bucky tray under the table: 60–75 kV, automatic, center cell
- Tabletop technique without Bucky: 55–70 kV; 4 mAs, __ mAs, __ mAs

▥ Patient Preparation

- Remove clothes from the waist down, except underwear
- Make certain that there is no fracture of the femur or lower leg (take a preliminary film if there are symptoms)

▲ Positioning

A. Knee AP (to test the medial and lateral ligaments)
- With the patient seated, the leg is flexed 15–30° (supported if necessary); the opposite leg is abducted
- The examiner, wearing lead apron and gloves, puts stress on the knee joint by applying lateral (or medial) traction on the foot, and with the other hand exerts pressure on the outside (or on the inside) of the knee joint
- If the restraining assembly is used, the pressure plate of the support is placed at the level of the joint space, exactly opposite the midpoint of the counterpressure pad, and pressure is set at 147 N (15 kp)
B. Lateral knee (to test the anterior and posterior cruciate ligaments)
- The patient lies on the affected side, with the lateral aspect of the knee down, knee flexed 90°. The examiner, wearing lead apron and gloves, holds the patient's leg parallel to the plane of the tabletop with one hand, and with the other hand (fist) exerts maximal pressure against the lower leg below the popliteal fossa ("anterior compartment"). When testing the anterior cruciate ligament ("posterior compartment"), the pressure is applied against the anterior surface of the lower leg while positioning remains otherwise the same
- When using restraining assembly, the knee is flexed 10–20° when placed into the holder, and pressure to be applied is set at 147 N (15 kp)

❗ Tips & Tricks

- Recheck pressure settings shortly before taking the films
- When testing the anterior cruciate ligament in muscular athletic patients, the pressure applied can be increased to 196 N (20 kp)

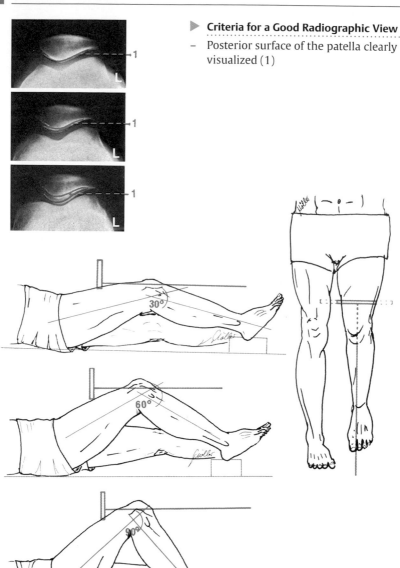

▶ **Criteria for a Good Radiographic View**

– Posterior surface of the patella clearly visualized (1)

◆ Imaging Technique

Image receiver (e.g., film): size 18×43 cm (7×17"), landscape, divided for three views on one film
Image receiver dosage (sensitivity class): ≤5 µGy (SC 400)
SID: 105 cm (40")
Bucky: no (tabletop technique)
Focal spot size: small (focal spot nominal value: ≤1.3)
Manual exposure: 50–60 kV; about 4 mAs, __ mAs, __ mAs

■ Patient Preparation

- Remove clothes from the waist down, except underwear

▲ Positioning

- Patient seated on the examining table
- Leg flexed:
  1st view: 150° (30°)
  2nd view: 120° (60°)
  3 rd view: 90° (90°)
  (angle of the longitudinal axis upper/lower leg)
- Patella parallel to the table
- Cassette placed upright on the thigh, perpendicular to the table (either in a cassette holder, or patients hold the cassette themselves)
- Upper border of the cassette = one hand's breadth above the patella
- Gonads shielded (large lead apron)

● Alignment

- Projection: horizontal caudocephalad (parallel to the patella)
- Central ray directed to the midpoint of the lower border of the patella, perpendicular to the middle of the cassette
- Centering, collimation, side identification

Variation

Patella, axial projection, Settegast position
- Prone position, thigh rests on the table, and the anterior knee on the cassette
- Lower leg flexed until upper and lower leg form an angle of 45°
- Projection and central ray as above

! Tips & Tricks

- For help with positioning, place cardboard cutouts (30°, 60°, 90°) at the side of the knee

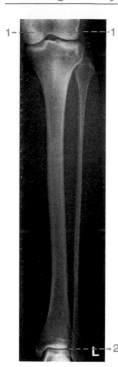

▶ **Criteria for a Good Radiographic View**

– Lower leg in straight AP projection
– Knee or ankle joint included on the film
– Femoral condyles form the lateral margins, patella superimposed on midfemur (1)
– Ankle joint clearly visualized (2)

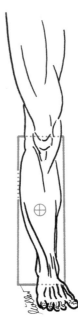

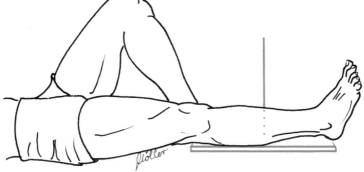

◆ **Imaging Technique**

Image receiver (e.g., film): size 18×43 cm (7×17"), portrait; or 30×40 cm (12×16"), divided; 20×40 cm (8×16") with knee joint, 15×20 cm (6×8") with ankle joint, with +/– compensating screen (+ towards the knee)
Image receiver dosage (sensitivity class): ≤5 μGy (SC 400)
SID: 115 cm (40") or 105 cm (40")
Bucky: yes (no)
Focal spot size: small (focal spot nominal value: ≤1.3)
Exposure:
    With Bucky tray under the table: 60–75 kV, automatic, center cell
–   Tabletop technique without Bucky:
    With knee joint: 50–70 kV; 4 mAs, __ mAs, __ mAs
    With ankle joint: 50–70 kV; 3–4 mAs, __ mAs, __ mAs

■ **Patient Preparation**
–   Remove clothes from the waist down, except underwear

▲ **Positioning**
–   Supine position, leg extended, slightly rotated medially:
A. with knee joint included: patella in frontal position
B. with ankle joint included: medial rotation, foot slightly dorsiflexed, opposite leg abducted
–   Cassette:
A. with knee joint: upper cassette border 4 cm above joint space
B. lower cassette border at the plantar level
–   Gonads shielded (large lead apron)

● **Alignment**
–   Projection: AP, perpendicular to the film
–   Central ray directed to the middle of the cassette
–   Centering, collimation, side identification

❗ **Tips & Tricks**
–   Put a bag with rice flour on the ankle joint and lower leg to compensate for density differences (compensating screen preferable)
–   To get a truly straight view of the joint of interest, center to the joint and angle the central ray to include the full field size
–   Maintain the rotation by immobilizing with a sandbag

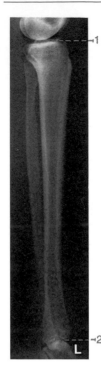

▶ **Criteria for a Good Radiographic View**

–   Lower leg straight lateral
–   Knee (1) or ankle joint (2) included on the film

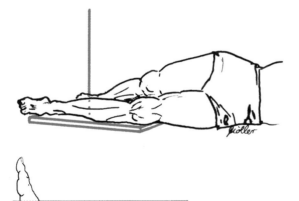

Lower Extremity

◆ Imaging Technique

Image receiver (e.g., film): size 18×43 cm (7×17"), portrait; or 30×40 cm (12×16"), divided; 20×40 cm (8×16") with knee joint, 15×20 cm (6×8") with ankle joint, with +/– compensating screen (+ towards the knee)

Image receiver dosage (sensitivity class): ≤5 µGy (SC 400)

SID: 115 cm (40") or 105 cm (40")

Bucky: yes (no)

Focal spot size: small (focal spot nominal value: ≤1.3)

Exposure:

– With Bucky tray under the table: 60–75 kV, automatic, center cell
– Tabletop technique without Bucky:
  With knee joint: 50–70 kV; 4 mAs, __ mAs, __ mAs
  With ankle joint: 50–70 kV; 3–4 mAs, __ mAs, __ mAs

▣ Patient Preparation

– Remove clothes from the waist down, except underwear

▲ Positioning

– Patient lying on side, knee flexed about 30°
– Outside of the lower leg parallel to the cassette
– Opposite leg placed behind the leg to be examined

Cassette:

A. with knee joint included: upper cassette border 4 cm above joint space, heel slightly supported
B. with ankle joint included: lower cassette border at plantar level, toes supported with a sponge wedge, foot slightly dorsiflexed
– Gonads shielded (large lead apron)

● Alignment

– Projection: mediolateral, perpendicular to the film
– Central ray directed to the middle of the cassette
– Centering, collimation, side identification

❗ Tips & Tricks

– Lateral position: lateral and medial malleolus in one plane
– Use compensating screen or rice flour, if necessary
– Take oblique views in 45° rotation, both medial and lateral

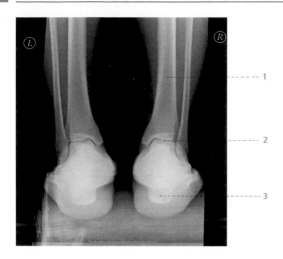

▶ **Criteria for a Good Radiographic View**

– Calcaneus (as for the axial view, 3), ankle (2) and lower leg (1) displayed.
Lower leg–calcaneus axis measurement possible.

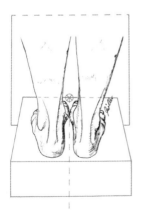

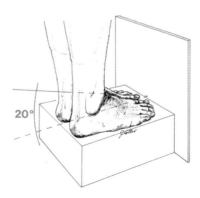

◆ Imaging Technique

Image receiver (e.g., film): size 35×43 cm (14×17") or 30×40 cm (12×16"), portrait, on vertical Bucky grid
Image receiver dosage (sensitivity class): ≤5 µGy (SC 400)
SID: 130 cm (50")
Bucky: no
Focal spot size: small (focal spot nominal value: 0.6 [≤1.3])
Manual exposure: 65 kV; 2.5 mAs, __ mAs, __ mAs

▦ Patient Preparation

- Uncover the leg

▲ Positioning

- Patient stands facing the vertical Bucky grid on a stable box that is permeable to röntgen rays
- Feet slightly apart
- Knee stretched but not straightened
- The vertical Bucky grid is moved downward as far as possible
- Gonads shielded (large lead apron)

● Alignment

- Projection: 20° craniocaudad
- Central ray directed to the ankle joint (at the level of the Achilles tendon)
- Centering, collimation, side identification (mirrored)

Advantages of the View

- This view is good for assessing the subtalar articular axis following calcaneal fractures.

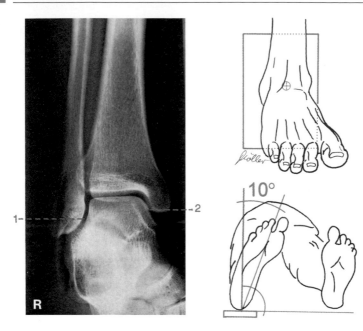

▶ **Criteria for a Good Radiographic View**

– Ankle joint completely visualized, including medial and lateral malleoli and distal fibula
– Joint space between the medial malleolus and the talus (inside, 2), and between the lateral malleolus and the talus (outside, 1) clearly visible

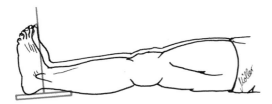

◆ Imaging Technique

Image receiver (e.g., film): size 18×24 cm (8×10"), landscape, divided for two views

Image receiver dosage (sensitivity class): ≤10 µGy (SC 200)

SID: 105 cm (40")

Bucky: no (tabletop technique)

Focal spot size: small (focal spot nominal value: ≤1.3)

Manual exposure: 50–60 kV; 4 mAs, __ mAs, __ mAs

■ Patient Preparation

– Uncover the lower leg

▲ Positioning

– Supine position, leg extended, foot slightly rotated medially, about 10–15°
– Foot dorsiflexed (plantar surface of the foot at a 90° angle with the lower leg)
– Opposite leg abducted
– Gonads shielded (large lead apron)

● Alignment

– Projection: AP, perpendicular to the film
– Central ray directed to the midpoint of the ankle joint (1 cm above the tip of the medial malleolus) and middle of the cassette
– Centering, collimation, side identification

! Tips & Tricks

– Check medial rotation of the foot by aligning the little toe with the center of the ankle joint
– Malleolar mortise parallel to the film (and at equal distance from the cassette)

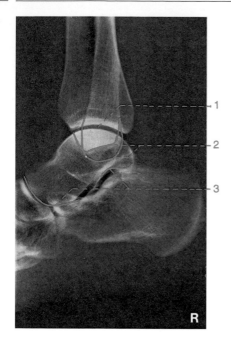

▶ **Criteria for a Good Radiographic View**

– Ankle joint (1) and talocalcaneonavicular joint (3) in true lateral projection (malleoli superimposed [2] on each other)
– Calcaneus and talus completely included in the view
– Fibula is projected over the middle to distal third of the tibial joint surface

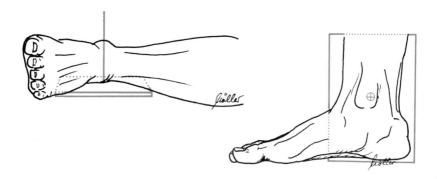

◆ Imaging Technique

Image receiver (e.g., film): size 18×24cm (8×10") landscape, divided for two views; or 18×24cm (8×10"), portrait
Image receiver dosage (sensitivity class): ≤10μGy (SC 200)
SID: 105cm (40")
Bucky: no (tabletop technique)
Focal spot size: small (focal spot nominal value: 0.6 [≤1.3])
Manual exposure: 50–60kV; 4mAs, __mAs, __mAs

■ Patient Preparation

– Uncover the lower leg

▲ Positioning

– Lateral position, the leg to be examined resting with the lateral malleolus close to the film
– Foot slightly dorsiflexed (lower leg/plantar surface = 90°)
– Straight lateral (malleoli exactly superimposed on each other)
– Flat sponge wedge put under the forefoot
– Healthy leg abducted
– Gonads shielded (large lead apron)

● Alignment

– Projection: mediolateral, perpendicular to the film
– Central ray directed to the center of the ankle joint (midpoint of the medial malleolus) and middle of the cassette
– Centering, collimation, side identification

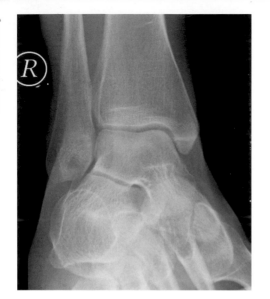

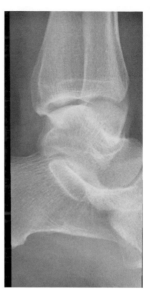

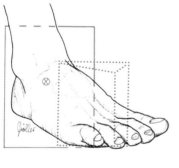

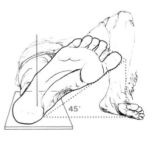

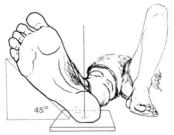

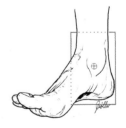

▶ **Criteria for a Good Radiographic View**

- View with internal rotation: good visualization of the posterior subtalar joint (3) and of the lateral ankle joint (2), with no superimposition of the lateral malleolus (1)
- View with external rotation: good depiction of the posterior edge of the tibia (4), with the fibula projected into the anterior section of the tibia (5)

◆ **Imaging Technique**

Image receiver (e.g., film): size 18×24 cm (8×10"), landscape, divided for two views; or 18×24 cm (8×10"), portrait
Image receiver dosage (sensitivity class): $\leq 10 \mu$Gy (SC 200)
SID: 105 cm (40")
Bucky: no (tabletop technique)
Focal spot size: small (focal spot nominal value: 0.6 [≤ 1.3])
Manual exposure: 50–60 kV; 10–16 mAs, __ mAs, __ mAs

■ **Patient Preparation**

- Uncover the lower leg

▲ **Positioning**

- Supine position, leg to be examined lying on table, contralateral leg angled (for support)
- Foot with heel lying on table, rotated 45° inward or outward (supported with 45° wedge cushion)
- Gonads shielded (large lead apron)

● **Alignment**

- Projection: AP
- Central ray directed to the midpoint of the ankle joint (1–2 cm above the tip of the medial malleolus or 2 3 cm above the tip of the lateral malleolus), perpendicular to the film at the middle of the film
- Centering, collimation, side identification
- Additional notation of 45° internal rotation or 45° external rotation

Advantages of the View

- This view is advantageous for fractures, particularly "flake" fractures of the trochlea of the talus or smaller fractures or avulsion injuries in the area of the syndesmosis. It is also good for supplementing the standard projections.

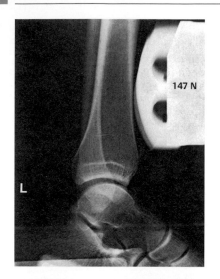

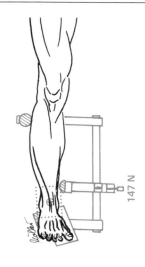

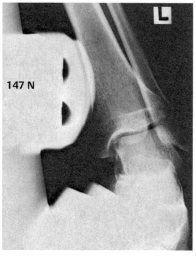

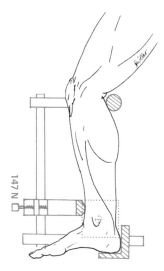

▶ **Criteria for a Good Radiographic View**
....

– Ankle joint completely visualized, including both malleoli
– Clear view of the joint mortise

❗ **Tips & Tricks**
....

– Recheck pressure settings shortly before taking the films

◆ **Imaging Technique**

Image receiver (e. g., film): size 18×24 cm (8 × 10"), landscape, divided for two views

Image receiver dosage (sensitivity class): ≤10 µGy (SC 200)

SID: 105 cm (40")

Bucky: no (tabletop technique)

Focal spot size: small (focal spot nominal value: ≤1.3)

Manual exposure: 50–60 kV, 4 mAs, __ mAs, __ mAs

▦ **Patient Preparation**

– Uncover the lower leg
– Rule out fracture (take a preliminary film if necessary)

▲ **Positioning**

A. As for AP ankle (to test the medial and lateral ligaments)
– Patient seated, leg bent 20° at knee (knee cushion)
– Contralateral leg abducted
– Foot is placed in restraining assembly (fix the heel in the foot-holder, upper support on exterior proximal lower leg, pressure plate of the support 1 FB above the medial malleolus = testing the exterior ligaments; vice versa for the interior ligaments)
– Set pressure to 147 N (15 kp)
B. As for lateral ankle (to test the anterior ligamentous support of the talus)
– Patient in lateral decubitus position, affected leg with the lateral malleolus downward (near the film)
– Foot slightly dorsiflexed (lower leg/plantar surface = 90°)
– Strictly lateral position (malleoli lying precisely superimposed)
– Contralateral leg abducted
– Foot is placed in restraining assembly (lower support at the heel, upper support on the calf approximately one hand's breadth below the knee joint, pressure plate of the support 2–3 FB above the medial malleolus from anterior onto the tibia)
– Set pressure to 147 N (15 kp), wait approximately 1 min before taking the film
– Gonads shielded (large lead apron)

● **Alignment**

– Projection: AP or lateral, perpendicular to the film
– Central ray directed to the midpoint of the ankle joint (1 cm above the tip of the medial malleolus) and to the middle of the cassette
– Centering, collimation, side identification, notation of applied pressure (147 N [15 kp])

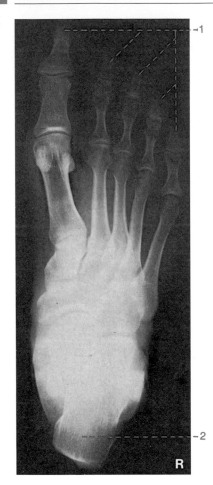

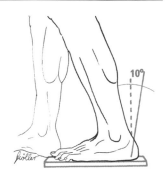

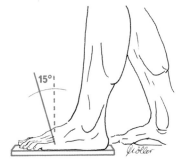

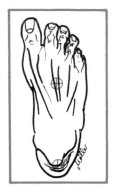

▶ **Criteria for a Good Radiographic View**

– Entire foot included, from the terminal phalanges (1) to the calcaneus (2) with no super-imposition

– Good exposure

◆ **Imaging Technique**

Image receiver (e.g., film): size 24×30 cm (10×12"), portrait
Image receiver dosage (sensitivity class): ≤10 μGy (SC 200 [SC 400]); if compensating screen is used, +/–, plus up)
SID: 105 cm (40")
Bucky: no (tabletop technique)
Focal spot size: small (focal spot nominal value: 0.6 [≤1.3])
Manual exposure: 50–60 kV; 4–6 mAs, __ mAs, __ mAs

▨ **Patient Preparation**

– Remove clothes from the waist down, except underwear

▲ **Positioning**

– Patient stands erect with the foot placed firmly on the cassette, which lies on the floor; foot immobilized on the cassette
– View 1: affected foot extended back as far as possible at the ankle joint, the opposite foot is placed for support behind the cassette, hands may grasp the armrest of a chair for additional support
– View 2: foot (with the plantar surface unchanged in its position) is anteflexed at the ankle joint; the opposite foot is placed in front of the cassette; hands may be placed for support on the thigh of the same side
– Gonads shielded (large lead aprons, one in front and one behind)

● **Alignment**

View 1
– Projection: 15° anterior oblique, dorsoplantar (or vertical)
– Central ray directed to the midfoot
View 2
– Projection: –10° posterior oblique, dorsoplantar
– Central ray directed to the mid-calcaneus
– Centering, collimation, side identification

❗ **Tips & Tricks**

– Use rice flour or a filter to compensate for density differences (except when there is possible primary chronic polyarthritis)

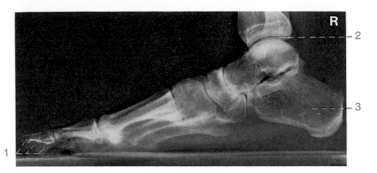

▶ **Criteria for a Good Radiographic View**

– Entire foot visible, including ankle joint (2), terminal phalanges (1), and calcaneus (3)
– Lateral projection of the ankle joint (2)

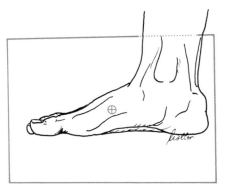

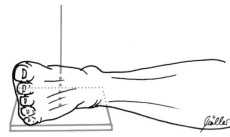

◆ **Imaging Technique**

Image receiver (e.g., film): size 24×30 cm (10×12"), landscape
Image receiver dosage (sensitivity class): ≤10 µGy (SC 200)
SID: 105 cm (40")
Bucky: no (tabletop technique)
Focal spot size: small (focal spot nominal value: 0.6 [≤1.3])
Manual exposure: 50–60 kV; 4–5 mAs, __ mAs, __ mAs

▦ **Patient Preparation**

– Uncover the foot (take off shoes, socks, pants)

▲ **Positioning**

– Patient lies on side on the examining table, small-toe side on the film
– Midfoot centered over the film
– Heel elevated with sponge wedge
– Knee with suitable support
– Opposite leg placed anteriorly
– Gonads shielded (large lead apron)

● **Alignment**

– Projection: mediolateral, perpendicular to the film
– Central ray directed to the midpoint of the foot and of the cassette
– Centering, collimation, side identification

Variations

– Examination may also be done with the patient standing up, a wooden block used for support, or in the supine position, a wooden block supporting the sole of the foot (at right angle to the axis of the lower leg)
– For small children, use a small board to dorsiflex the foot as far as possible (to demonstrate club foot)

Lower Extremity

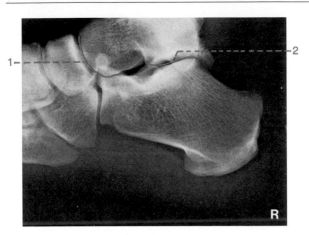

▶ **Criteria for a Good Radiographic View**

– True lateral projection
– Calcaneus completely visualized
– Talocalcaneonavicular joint (1 and 2) clearly demonstrated

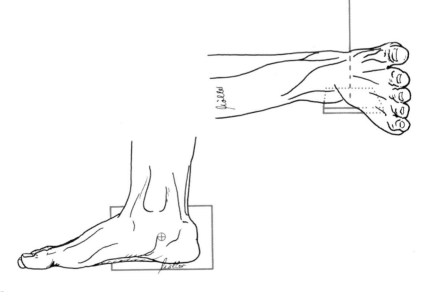

Lower Extremity

◆ Imaging Technique

Image receiver (e. g., film): size 13 × 18 cm (5 × 7"), landscape; or 18 × 24 cm (8 × 10"), landscape, divided for two views)
Image receiver dosage (sensitivity class): ≤ 10 µGy (SC 200)
SID: 105 cm (40")
Bucky: no (tabletop technique)
Focal spot size: small (focal spot nominal value: 0.6 [≤ 1.3])
Manual exposure: 50–60 kV; 4 mAs, __ mAs, __ mAs

▨ Patient Preparation

– Uncover thee foot (take off shoes, socks, pants)

▲ Positioning

– Patient lies on side to be examined, lateral (small toe) side on the film
– Heel supported (elevated about 10–15°)
– Leg flexed at the hip and knee
– The opposite leg placed anteriorly
– Heel centered over the cassette
– Gonads shielded (large lead apron)

● Alignment

– Projection: mediolateral, perpendicular to the film
– Central ray directed to the calcaneus (2–3 cm below and behind the medial malleolus) and to the center of the film
– Centering, collimation, side identification

❗ Tips & Tricks

– To evaluate the Achilles tendon (for possible rupture), use a softer beam (35–40 kV)

Lower Extremity

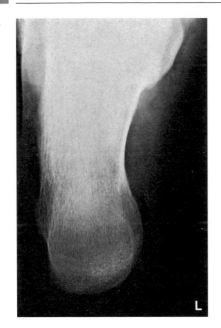

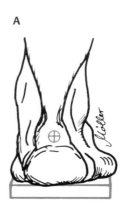

A

▶ **Criteria for a Good Radiographic View**
- Posterior aspect of the calcaneus clearly visible
- Calcaneus complete and unforeshortened

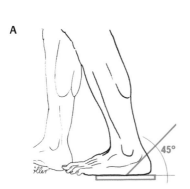

A

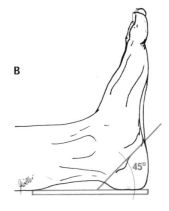

B

◆ **Imaging Technique**

Image receiver (e.g., film): size 13×18 cm (5×7"), portrait
Image receiver dosage (sensitivity class): ≤10 μGy (SC 200)
SID: 105 cm (40")
Bucky: no (tabletop technique)
Focal spot size: small (focal spot nominal value: 0.6 [≤1.3])
Manual exposure: 50–60 kV; 4 mAs, __ mAs, __ mAs

■ **Patient Preparation**

– Uncover the foot (take off shoes, socks, pants)

▲ **Positioning**

– A. Patient places the foot on the cassette, foot flexed at the ankle joint
– B. Supine position, foot dorsiflexed (toes pulled with a hand towards the lower leg as far as possible, foot and lower leg are in one plane = slight medial rotation), heel resting on the cassette (lower cassette border)
– Gonads shielded (large lead apron)

● **Alignment**

– Projection: A, 45° oblique dorsoplantar; B, 45° oblique plantodorsal
– Central ray directed to the midpoint of the calcaneus and center of the film
– Centering, collimation, side identification

❗ **Tips & Tricks**

– Use rice flour to compensate for differences in density to provide good visualization of detail also of the anterior parts of the calcaneus, then use about 55 kV

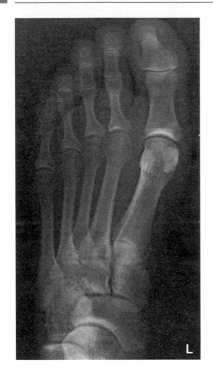

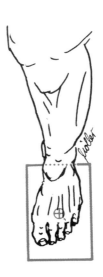

▶ **Criteria for a Good Radiographic View**

– Complete view of the forefoot (and midfoot) without any superimposition

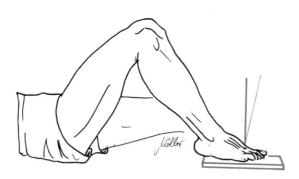

◆ **Imaging Technique**

Image receiver (e.g., film): size 18×24 cm (8×10"), landscape, divided for two views

Image receiver dosage (sensitivity class): ≤10 μGy (SC 200)

SID: 105 cm (40")

Bucky: no (tabletop technique)

Focal spot size: small (focal spot nominal value: 0.6 [≤1.3])

Manual exposure: 50–60 kV; 3–4 mAs, __ mAs, __ mAs

▪ **Patient Preparation**

– Uncover the foot (take off shoes, socks, pants)

▲ **Positioning**

– Patient sits on the X-ray table, leg pulled up, forefoot and midfoot stand with their plantar surface on the cassette
– Gonads shielded (large lead apron)

● **Alignment**

– Projection: perpendicular to the middle of the film (or 10° caudocephalad)
– Central ray directed to the head of the 3rd metatarsal (or to the midportion of the 3rd metatarsal if the midfoot is to be included) and to the center of the film
– Centering, collimation, side identification

Variation

View of the toes without any superimposition

– Image receiver (e.g., film): size 13×18 cm (5×7")
– Manual exposure: 40 kV; 8 mAs, __ mAs, __ mAs
– Otherwise as above
– Patient in prone position on the examining table
– The foot is rotated inward and rests with the back of the toes on the cassette
– Supported with a sponge wedge

❗ **Tips & Tricks**

– Use compensation filter or rice flour bag as needed
– Separate the toes with small rolled-up gauze pads or cotton balls

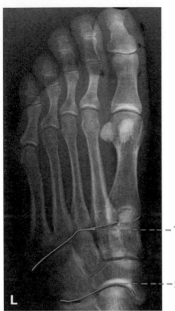

─ 1

─ 2

L

▶ **Criteria for a Good Radiographic View**

– Complete visualization of the forefoot and midfoot without any significant superimposition
– Clear demonstration of the Lisfranc (tarsometatarsal) (1) and Chopart (mediotarsal) (2) joints

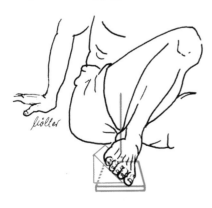

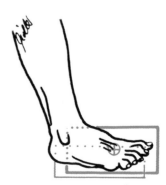

◆ **Imaging Technique**

Image receiver (e.g., film): size 24×30 cm (10×12"), landscape, divided for two views

Image receiver dosage (sensitivity class): ≤10 μGy (SC 200)

SID: 105 cm (40")

Bucky: no (tabletop technique)

Focal spot size: small (focal spot nominal value: 0.6 [≤1.3])

Manual exposure:

- Forefoot, oblique: 50–60 kV; 3–4 mAs, __ mAs, __ mAs
- Foot (midfoot and forefoot), oblique: 50–60 kV; 4 mAs, __ mAs, __ mAs
- Compensating filter if necessary

▨ **Patient Preparation**

- Uncover the foot (take off shoes, socks, pants)

▲ **Positioning**

- Patient sits on the X-ray table, leg drawn up, foot (forefoot) rests on the cassette
- Lower leg (and foot) adducted 45° (small-toe side elevated 45° and supported with a sponge wedge)
- Gonads shielded (large lead apron)

● **Alignment**

- Projection: perpendicular to the middle of the film
- Central ray directed to, either
  (a) head of the 3rd metatarsal (forefoot) and middle of the film, or
  (b) midportion of the 3rd metatarsal (forefoot- and midfoot) and middle of the film
- Centering, collimation, side identification

❗ **Tips & Tricks**

- Separate the toes with small gauze pads

Lower Extremity

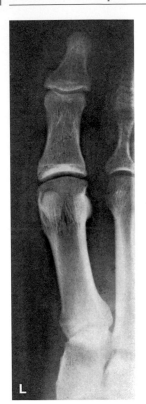

▶ **Criteria for a Good Radiographic View**
....
– Great toe completely visualized with no superimposition

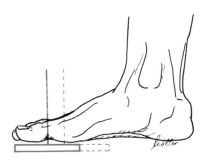

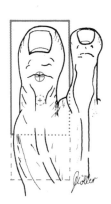

◆ **Imaging Technique**

Image receiver (e.g., film): size 13×18 cm (5×7"), portrait, divided for two views

Image receiver dosage (sensitivity class): $\leq 10 \mu$Gy (SC 200)

SID: 105 cm (40")

Bucky: no (tabletop technique)

Focal spot size: small (focal spot nominal value: 0.6 [≤ 1.3])

Manual exposure: 50–60 kV; 2 mAs, __ mAs, __ mAs

■ **Patient Preparation**

- Uncover the foot (take off shoes, socks)

▲ **Positioning**

- Patient sits on the X-ray table, leg drawn up, the great toe rests flat on the cassette
- Padding (cotton) between the 1st and 2nd toes
- Gonads shielded (large lead apron)

● **Alignment**

- Projection: dorsoplantar, perpendicular to the middle of the film
- Central ray directed to the metacarpophalangeal joint of the great toe and middle of the film
- Centering, collimation to terminal phalanx or great toe, side identification

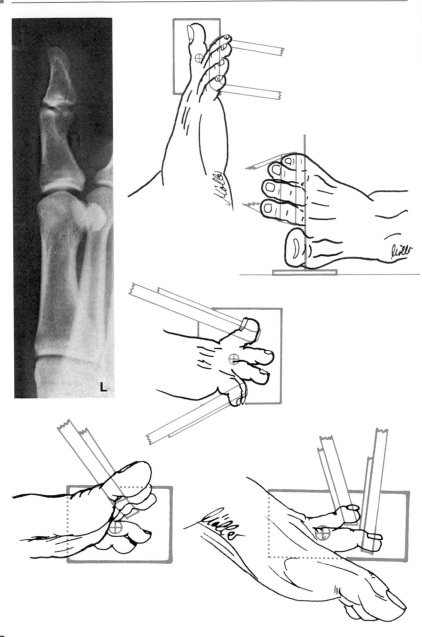

▶ **Criteria for a Good Radiographic View**
- Toe visualized in true lateral projection

◆ **Imaging Technique**
Image receiver (e.g., film): size 13 × 18 cm (5 × 7"), portrait, divided for two views
Image receiver dosage (sensitivity class): ≤ 10 µGy (SC 200)
SID: 105 cm (40")
Bucky: no (tabletop technique)
Focal spot size: small (focal spot nominal value: 0.6 [< 1.3])
Manual exposure: 50–60 kV; 2–3 mAs, __ mAs, __ mAs

▨ **Patient Preparation**
- Uncover the foot (take off shoes, socks)

▲ **Positioning**
Toes 1–3
- Patient lies on the unaffected side, the great toe is placed laterally on the cassette
- (a) Great toe: the 2nd to 5th toes are pulled down with a band (strip of bandage)
- (b) Toes 2 and 3: the great toe is pulled up with a band, 4th and 5th toes are pulled down
Toes 4 and 5
- Patient lies on the affected side, the little toe is placed laterally on the cassette
- Either toes 4 and 5 are elevated separately with a band each, or toes 1–3 are pulled up together
- Gonads shielded (large lead apron)

● **Alignment**
- Projection: mediolateral or lateromedial, perpendicular to the middle of the film
- Central ray directed to the metatarsophalangeal joint and midpoint of the film
- Centering, collimation, side identification

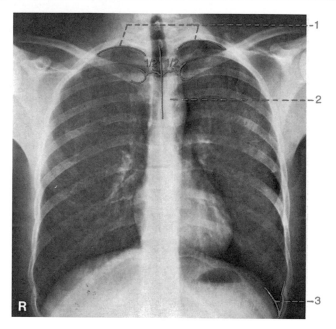

▶ **Criteria for a Good Radiographic View**

- Lungs fully visualized (apex of the lung [1] and costophrenic angle [3] clearly visible)
- Symmetrical depiction of the chest (heads of the clavicles equidistant from the spinous processes, spine [2] centered)
- Sharp view

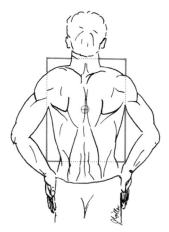

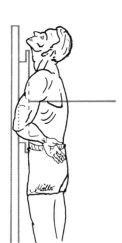

◆ **Imaging Technique**

Image receiver (e.g., film): size 40×40 cm (16×15"), portrait
Image receiver dosage (sensitivity class): ≤5 µGy (SC 400)
SID: 180–200 cm (70–80")
Bucky: yes (cassette stand; under the table, r 12 [8])
Focal spot size: small (large in obese patients) (focal spot nominal value: ≤1.3)
Exposure: 125 kV; automatic, right lateral cell

■ **Patient Preparation**

- Remove all clothes from the waist up
- Take off jewelry (necklace, earrings)
- Tie back hair

▲ **Positioning**

- Patient stands with the chest facing the vertical cassette stand, leaning slightly forward
- Chest wall and both shoulders in contact with the cassette (patient lets the shoulders hang down)
- Hands placed on the hips, elbows rotated forward
- Head extended with the chin over the top of the cassette
- Upper cassette border 3 FB above the upper border of the shoulder
- Gonads shielded (lead apron)

● **Alignment**

- Projection: dorsoventral (PA), perpendicular to the film
- Central ray directed to the spinal column at the level of the lower pole of the scapula
- Centering, collimation to the skin surface of the inferior costal arches, side identification
- Breath held after deep inspiration

Variation

Chest in the recumbent position
- Manual exposure: 90–110 kV; __ mAs, __ mAs, __ mAs
- Bucky: 8/40 grid
If pneumothorax is suspected: additional view after expiration

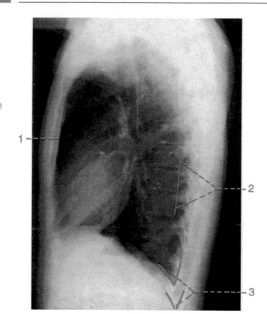

▶ **Criteria for a Good Radiographic View**

– Lungs completely visualized (costophrenic angles clearly visible, 3)
– Sternum on the lateral margin (no rips superimposed in front of the sternum, 1)
– Posterior edges of the vertebrae with clear contours (2)

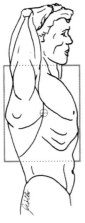

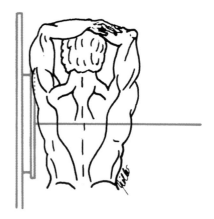

◆ Imaging Technique

Image receiver (e. g., film): size 30×40 cm (12×16") or 40×40 cm (16×16") or 35×43 cm (14×17"), portrait
Image receiver dosage (sensitivity class): ≤5 µGy (SC 400)
SID: 180–200 cm (70–80")
Bucky: yes (cassette stand; under the table, r 12 [8])
Focal spot size: large (focal spot nominal value: ≤1.3)
Exposure: 125 kV, automatic, center cell

■ Patient Preparation

– Remove all clothes from the waist up
– Take off jewelry (necklace, earrings)
– Tie back hair

▲ Positioning

– Patient stands erect, with the left side against the film, straight lateral
– Arms extended upward above the head (or forehead, hands grasp the elbows)
– Upper body leans slightly forward
– Upper cassette border 3 FB above the upper border of the shoulder (vertebra prominens = 7th cervical vertebra)
– Gonads shielded (lead apron)

● Alignment

– Projection: lateral, perpendicular to the film
– Central ray directed to the anterior axillary line at the level of the nipple (or tip of the sternum)
– Centering, collimation, side identification

Variation

– Right lateral view only in special diagnostic situations

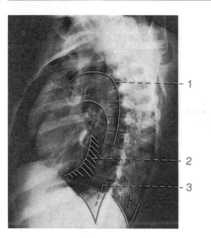
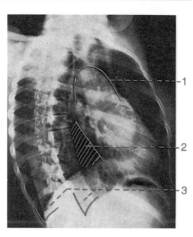

▶ **Criteria for a Good Radiographic View**
....

- A. Aortic arch uncoiled (1), retrocardiac space clearly visible (cardiac shadow projected away from the vertebral column, 2), lungs included from the apex to the costophrenic angle (3)
- B. Aortic arch foreshortened (1), retrocardiac space clearly visible (cardiac shadow projected away from the vertebral column, 2), esophagus demonstrated without any superimposition, lungs included from the apex to the costophrenic angle (3)

First oblique
(RAO)
position
(fencer
position)

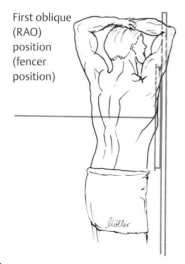

Second oblique
(RAO)
position
(boxer
position)

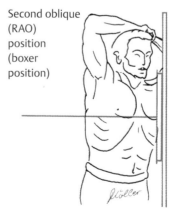

◆ **Imaging Technique**

Image receiver (e.g., film): size 35×43 cm (14×17") or 40×40 cm (16×16") or 35×35 cm (17×17")
Image receiver dosage (sensitivity class): ≤5 µGy (SC 400)
SID: 180–200 cm (70–80")
Bucky: yes (under the table, vertical Bucky, r 12 [8])
Focal spot size: large (focal spot nominal value: ≤1.3)
Exposure: 125 kV, automatic, lateral cells

■ **Patient Preparation**

– Remove all clothes from the waist up
– Take off jewelry (necklace, earrings)
– Tie back hair

▲ **Positioning**

– A. First oblique (RAO, fencer position): patient stands at an oblique angle
   of 45° (to 60°) toward the plane of the film, right anterior chest wall in
   contact with the upright cassette
– B. Second oblique (LAO, boxer position): patient stands at an oblique angle
   of 45° (to 35°) toward the plane of the film, left anterior chest wall in
   contact with the upright cassette
– Arms raised above the head
– Upper border of the cassette 3 FB above the upper border of the shoulder
– Gonads shielded (small lead apron)

● **Alignment**

– Projection: oblique dorsoventral, perpendicular to the film
– Central ray directed to the vertebral column (not to the line of spinous
   processes but about one hand's breadth beside the processes) at the level
   of the inferior angle of the scapula
– Centering, collimation to skin border, side identification

! **Tips & Tricks**

– A contrast swallow may be used to outline the posterior cardiac border

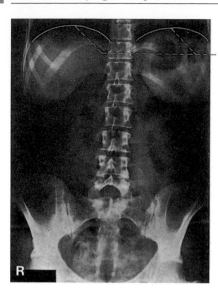

▶ **Criteria for a Good Radiographic View**

– Both domes of the diaphragm (1) and, as far as possible, the entire abdomen visualized completely and symmetrically

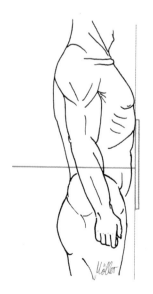

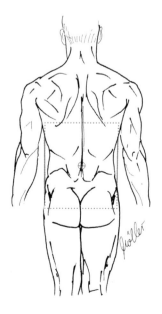

◆ Imaging Technique

Image receiver (e.g., film): size 35×43 cm (14×17"), portrait
Image receiver dosage (sensitivity class): ≤5 µGy (SC 400)
SID: 115 cm (40")
Bucky: yes (under the table, vertical Bucky, r 12 [8])
Focal spot size: large (focal spot nominal value ≤1.3)
Exposure: 100–125 kV, automatic, both exterior cells

▨ Patient Preparation

– Undress completely

▲ Positioning

– Patient stands upright, the anterior abdomen against the vertical grid
– Upper cassette border at the level of the xiphoid process
– Gonads shielded (testicle cups for males)

● Alignment

– Projection: dorsoventral, perpendicular to the film
– Central ray directed to the spinal column 1 FB above the iliac wing, middle of the cassette
– Collimation at least to the skin border or to $^1/_2$ FB less than film size
– Side identification and "upright" marker
– Breath held after expiration

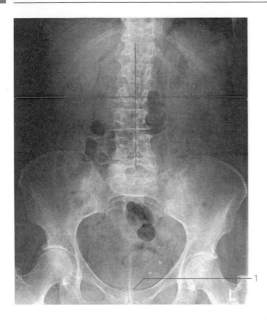

▶ **Criteria for a Good Radiographic View**

- Upper border of the symphysis (1) demonstrated (also the domes of the diaphragms, if possible)
- Spinal column in midline position (2)

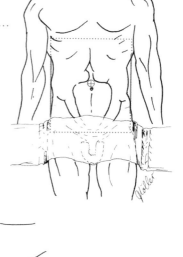

Other Noncontrast Diagnostic Studies

◆ Imaging Technique

Image receiver (e.g., film): size 35 × 43 cm (14 × 17"), portrait
Image receiver dosage (sensitivity class): ≤5 µGy (SC 400)
SID: 115 cm (40")
Bucky: yes (under the table, r 12 [8])
Focal spot size: large (focal spot nominal value ≤1.3)
Exposure: 80–90 kV, automatic, both exterior cells

■ Patient Preparation

– Undress completely

▲ Positioning

– Supine position, arms along the sides of the body
– Lower cassette border 1 FB below the upper border of the symphysis
– Gonads shielded (testicle cups for men)

● Alignment

– Projection: ventrodorsal, perpendicular to the film
– Central ray directed to mid-cassette in median plane, about 1 FB above the pelvic crest
– Lateral collimation to the anterior superior iliac spine on both sides
– Side identification and "supine" marker
– Breath held after expiration

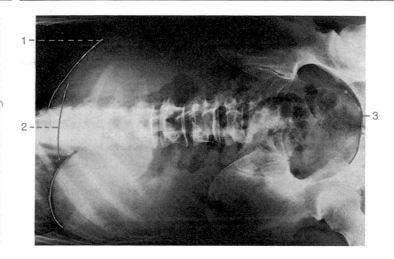

▶ **Criteria for a Good Radiographic View**

— Correct exposure of the entire abdomen, especially of the right costo-phrenic space (1)
— The entire abdomen, from the diaphragm (2) to the upper border of the pubic symphysis (3), is included in the film

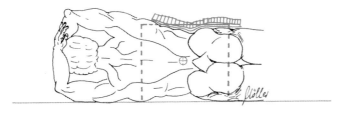

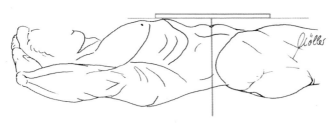

◆ Imaging Technique

Image receiver (e.g., film): size 35×43 cm (14×17"), portrait
Image receiver dosage (sensitivity class): ≤5 µGy (SC 400)
SID: 115 cm (40")
Bucky: yes (vertical Bucky grid, r 12 [8])
Focal spot size: large (focal spot nominal value ≤1.3)
Exposure: 100–125 kV, automatic, center cell (–1)

▧ Patient Preparation

– Undress completely

▲ Positioning

– Patient lies with the back (or abdomen in obese patients) against the cassette
– Arms placed above the head, legs slightly flexed for stabilization (patient must have been lying on the left side for at least 5 min to give possible free air time to rise)
– Upper border of the cassette 1 FB above the xiphoid process
– Attach a marker stating "right lateral decubitus" or "left lateral decubitus"
– Breath held after expiration
– Gonads shielded (testicle cups for men)

● Alignment

– Projection: ventrodorsal (or dorsoventral), horizontal, perpendicular to the film
– Central ray directed to the spinal column 2 FB above the iliac crest and middle of the cassette
– Use of a filter to compensate for differences in density
– Collimation at least to the skin border, or to $^1/_2$ FB less than film size
– Side identification and marker stating "left decubitus" or "right decubitus"
– Breath held after expiration

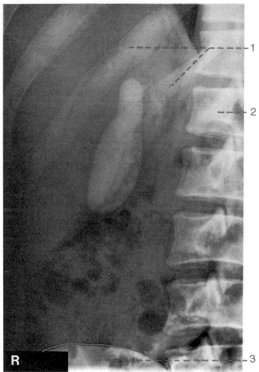

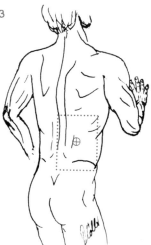

▶ **Criteria for a Good Radiographic View**

- Lowest rib (1) and iliac crest (3) are both visualized
- Spinal column (2) projected along the film edge

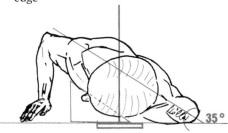

Other Noncontrast Diagnostic Studies

◆ **Imaging Technique**

Image receiver (e.g., film): size 24×30 cm (10×12"), portrait
Image receiver dosage (sensitivity class): ≤5 µGy (SC 400)
SID: 115 cm (40")
Bucky: yes (under the table, r 12 [8])
Focal spot size: large (focal spot nominal value ≤1.3)
Exposure: 70–80 kV, automatic, center cell

■ **Patient Preparation**

– Undress, except underwear

▲ **Positioning**

– Patient in the prone position, right side elevated about 35° (20–45°), supported with a sponge wedge (left arm along the side of the body, the right arm used for support, knees slightly flexed for additional stability)
– Right side of the body (midpoint between lowest rib and iliac crest) centered over the cassette
– Gonads shielded

● **Alignment**

– Projection: oblique ventrodorsal, perpendicular to the film
– Central ray directed to the middle of the cassette (about a hand's breadth lateral to the spinous processes, at the midpoint between the lowest rib and the iliac crest)
– Centering, lateral collimation to the skin border, side identification
– Breath held after expiration

Variation

If tomographic films of the gallbladder are needed:
– 70 kV, medium thickness of the tomographic slices, at a depth of 8–12 cm

❗ **Tips & Tricks**

Mark the central ray on the skin with a skin marker (for later films or corrections)
– Obese patient: gallbladder (and film center) more cranial and lateral (20° elevation is sufficient)
– Thin patient: gallbladder (and film center) lower in the pelvis and more medial (elevation of the right side up to 45°)

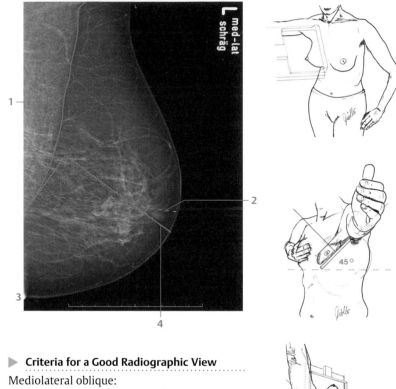

▶ **Criteria for a Good Radiographic View**

Mediolateral oblique:
- The pectoral muscle should appear as a tri-angle (with an angle of about 20°) (1)
- The pectoral muscle extends to the level of the nipple (the posterior nipple line can be used for guidance—an imaginary line connecting the nipple and the anterior edge of the pectoral muscle) (2)
- Nipple tangential outside the breast tissue
- Inframammary fold shown spread out (3)
- The distance from the nipple to the pectoral muscle on the pectoral–nipple line (PNL; a vertical line connecting the edge of the pectoral muscle and the nipple [4]) should vary not more than ± 1.5 cm from the distance on the PNL in the craniocaudal image

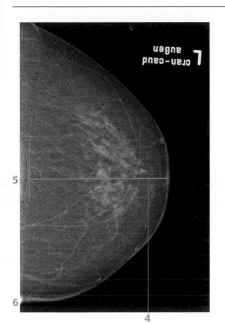

▶ **Criteria for a Good Radiographic View**

Craniocaudal
- Pectoral muscle should be crescent-shaped at the edge of the image (5)
- Retroglandular fatty tissue should be well displayed
- Medial fold displayed (6)
- Nipple tangential outside the breast tissue
- Entire breast (including medial) displayed
- The distance from the nipple to the pectoral muscle on the pectoral–nipple line (PNL; a vertical line connecting the edge of the pectoral muscle and the nipple [4]) should vary not more than ± 1.5 cm from the distance on the PNL in the mediolateral image

Other Noncontrast Diagnostic Studies

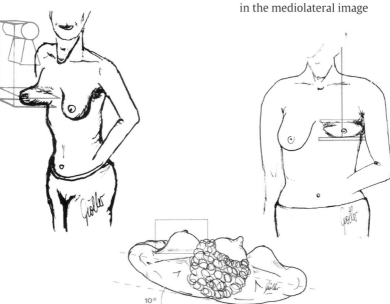

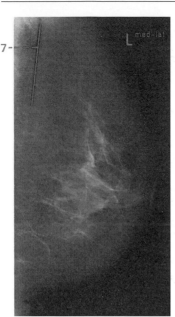

7-

▶ **Criteria for a Good Radiographic View**

Mediolateral
- Entire breast (including medial) should be displayed with no superimposition (not "hanging")
- The axillary fold should have no superimposition
- The pectoral muscle should be a very narrow wedge up to about the level of the nipple (7)
- Nipple tangential outside the breast tissue
- Inferior fold stretched

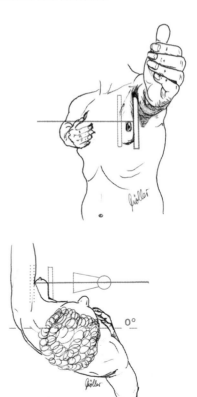

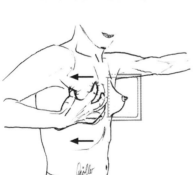

◆ **Imaging Technique**

Image receiver (e.g., special one-sided film): size 18×24 cm (8×10")
Image receiver dosage corresponds to EK 25 (nominal dosage: analogue to KN ≤100 μGy)
SID: ≥60 cm, with special device ≥55 cm
Bucky: yes (mobile special grid r 4, 27 L/cm; r 5, 30 L/cm)
Focal spot nominal value: ≤0.3, digital ≤0.4; for magnification technique, microfocus 0.1 mm possible
Exposure: 25–35 kV relative to diameter and density
Automatic exposure: cell position specially adjustable, good adjustment for diameter, density, and tube voltage
Exposure time: <2 s
(Compression ≥10 kp)

▦ **Patient Preparation**

– Remove clothes from the waist up, remove jewelry

▲ **Positioning**

Mediolateral oblique (MLO)
– The imaging unit is rotated 45–60° depending on the course of the pectoral muscle (the lateral edge of the pectoral muscle should run parallel to the supporting table)
– The patient stands obliquely at an angle of about 45° to the device. The supporting table is raised to the level of the axilla under the anterior axillary fold.
– The arm on the side being examined lies relaxed on the cassette holder or detector.
– The breast is raised and drawn anteriorly away from the chest wall in the direction of the nipple. As compression proceeds, the breast should be smoothed out in the direction of the nipple without folds, and the breast tissue should be well spread. The nipple remains in a tangential position.
– The long side of the compression paddle should be firmly against the sternum
– The patient holds the contralateral breast away from the projection
Craniocaudal (CC)
– The imaging unit is positioned horizontally at about the level of the inframammary fold.
– The patient stands upright, turned about 10° medially and about 5 cm away from the imaging unit (so that she can lean forward slightly into the device afterward)

- The head is turned toward the contralateral side.
- The shoulder is loose, and the arm on the side being examined lies relaxed on the abdomen.
- The patient's breast should be raised to the limit of its natural mobility and the imaging unit should be placed in its final position
- The nipple lies in a tangential position in the center (more medially)
- The breast is drawn anteriorly away from the chest wall (the patient's back should be supported during compression to prevent recoil movement).
- The photocells are placed in a retromammillary position in the anterior two-thirds.

Mediolateral (ML), lateromedial (LM)

- The imaging unit is positioned vertically.
- The patient stands leaning forward slightly directly in front of the cassette holder or detector, with the outer side of the breast (mediolateral) or inner side (lateromedial) facing the cassette
- The arm on the side being examined lies relaxed on the cassette holder or detector
- The corner of the imaging unit lies directly in the axillary fossa
- The breast is carefully raised from the inferior fold, drawn forward, and smoothed out (the breast is supported until the end of the compression process)
- The nipple is tangential and at the center of the film
- The patient holds the contralateral breast away from the projection

For all images:

- Side and projection (MLO, CC, or ML or LM) should be noted on the exposure
- Gonads shielded

● **Alignment**
....
- Projection: perpendicular to the film (MLO, CC, or ML or LM)
- Breath held

Variations
....
Axillary projection (similar to the alignment for the MLO view)

- Specific indication: enlarged lymph nodes or tumor infiltration in the axillary fossa

Position

- The imaging unit is rotated 45–60°, depending on the course of the pectoral muscle
- The patient stands slightly obliquely towards the device

- The supporting table is raised to the level of the axilla, underneath the anterior axillary fold
- The arm on the side being examined is stretched out horizontally
- The upper part of the breast with the extended axilla is positioned well onto the imaging unit, so that the anterior axillary fold can be well compressed
- The patient holds the contralateral breast away from the projection

Alignment
- Projection: ventrodorsal
- Central ray directed toward the center of the anterior axillary fold in the middle of the cassette
- Photocells: near the chest wall
- Side label and axilla (AX) should be exposed on the film
- Imaging with breath held

Cleopatra view:
- Specific indication: imaging of the lateral quadrant of the breast in CC projection

Position
- Imaging unit perpendicular or angled 5°
- The patient stands slightly obliquely in front of the imaging unit, with the side being examined at the front
- The patient leans well to the side and backward (pushes the lateral quadrant forward onto the imaging unit)
- Nipple tangential, pointing clearly toward the center

Alignment
- Projection: craniocaudal oblique
- Central ray directed toward the exterior quadrants in the middle of the cassette
- Photocells: retromammillary in the anterior two-thirds
- Side label and CC should be exposed on the film
- Imaging with breath held

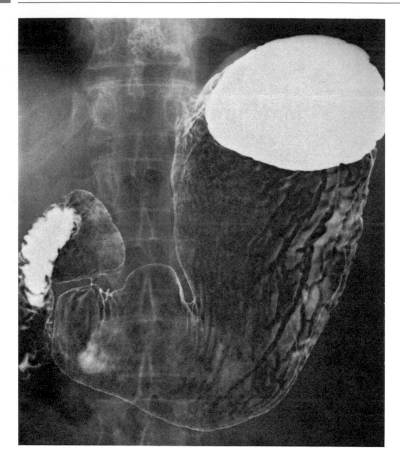

Patient Preparation

– Patient fasting; avoids nicotine

Materials and Radiographic Technique

– Cup of high-density contrast material (approx. 200 g barium sulfate/ 100 mL or oral Micropaque)
– Drinking cup for the contrast (about 150–220 mL)
– Drinking cup with about 10–15 mL water

- Bag with CO_2 granules (or 1 heaped teaspoon of effervescent powder [about 300 mL air])
- 18-gauge needle
- 2 mL syringe with 2 mL hyoscine butylbromide (Buscopan) (20 mg) (caution: glaucoma and tachycardia) or
- Insulin syringe with 15 graduations = 0.4 mg glucagon
- Skin preparation, sponges, tourniquet
- Image receiver system (e.g. film sizes: two 18 × 24 cm (8 × 10"), three 24 × 30 cm (10 × 12") films
- Exposure: 100–110 kV, automatic, center cell
  Focal spot nominal value: ≤ 1.3 (0.6)
- Bucky: r 8
- *Image receiver dosage* (sensitivity class): ≤ 5 µGy (SC 400)
- Object–detector distance: as small as possible
- Starting position for the fluoro unit: upright
- All films are taken in expiration

Examination Technique

- Injection of Buscopan or glucagon (supine)
- One swallow of contrast material (about 16–20 mL)

1st film: anterior wall/rugal relief pattern
- Prone position; 18 × 24 cm (8 × 10"), landscape
- Have patient drink the rest of the contrast (leave enough for one swallow) in upright position
- Observe the esophagus

2nd film: fill-up views of the distended stomach (the lesser curvature is projected free, rapid examination is necessary)
- Upright position; 24 × 30 cm (10 × 12"), portrait
- Have patient drink the effervescent powder with water
- Turn patient on left side and tilt table horizontally
- Have patient turn from the left lateral position onto the abdomen, then turn left again over onto back
- This procedure should be repeated three times in order to get good contrast coating
- If the patient has difficulties turning, have him or her make rocking motions lying on the left side
- Finally, have patient turn slowly to the right side and onto the stomach, then to the left side (if the coating is poor, the procedure should be repeated)

3 rd film: double-contrast view
– Supine position: 24 × 30 cm (10 × 12"), landscape (or portrait)
4th film: double-contrast spot films
– Have patient turn from the left side onto back; 24 × 30 cm (10 × 12"), land-scape, divided for four spot views
1st exposure: antrum with pylorus, duodenal bulb
2nd exposure: gastric angle and lower body region
3 rd exposure: upper body and gastric fundus with hiatal junction
(Schatzki position), patient turned slightly to the right side, table tilted
45° (the contrast material flows into the antrum and back to the cardia)
Check for hiatal hernia in this position:
– Have patient take a swallow of the contrast material, then tilt the table to lower the head
– Prone position, left side slightly elevated, have patient bear down. If find-ings are abnormal:
4th exposure: esophageal hiatus hernia
or
4th exposure: gastric fundus and cardia (upright)
5th film: compression spot films
– Upright; 18 × 24 cm (8 × 10"), landscape, divided into four spots, compres-sion cone
1st exposure: antrum
2nd exposure: greater curvature
3 rd exposure: duodenal bulb
4th exposure: varies, e. g., lesser curvature, duodenal bulb

Variations

First variation in examining technique
If the duodenal bulb does not unfold during the first exposure (together with the antrum), it can be rechecked later during the series of films. Between 4th and 5th films (even with hiatal hernia), take an additional
6th film:
– 18 × 24 cm (8 × 10"), landscape, divided for two views
For example:
1st view: fundus and cardia
2nd view: duodenal bulb
Then continued with the 5th film: compression views (see above)

Second variation in examining technique
Start out right away with double-contrast views:
– Materials and technique as above
– Films: two 18×24 cm (8×10"), two 24×30 cm (10×12")
1st film: double-contrast view
– Supine position; 24×30 cm (10×12"), landscape (or portrait)
2nd film: double-contrast spot films
– Have patient turn from the left side onto the back; 24×30 cm (10×12"),
  landscape, divided for four spot views
  1st exposure: antrum with pylorus, duodenal bulb
  2nd exposure: gastric angle and lower body region
  3rd exposure: upper body and gastric fundus with hiatal junction
  (Schatzki position), patient turned slightly to the right side, table tilted
  45° (the contrast material flows into the antrum and back to the cardia)
Check for hiatal hernia in this position:
– Have patient take a swallow of the contrast material, then tilt the table to
  lower the head
– Prone position, left side slightly elevated, have patient bear down. If findings are abnormal:
  4th exposure: esophageal hiatus hernia
  or
  4th exposure: gastric fundus and cardia (upright)
3rd film: fill-up view of the stomach (lesser curvature projected free)
Upright position; 24×30 cm (10×12"), portrait
4th film: compression spot films
Upright position; 18×24 cm (8×10"), landscape, divided into four views, compression cone
  1st exposure: antrum
  2nd exposure: greater curvature
  3rd exposure: duodenal bulb
  4th exposure: varies, e.g., lesser curvature, bulb

Variations depending on indication
– If there is a question of gastric outlet obstruction, perforation, or foreign
  body, use iodinated contrast medium
– Films as needed, at least one 24×30 cm (10×12") survey film, in some
  cases 18×24 cm (8×10"), landscape, divided in two

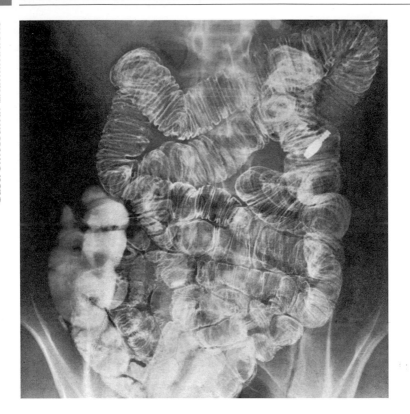

Patient Preparation

- Laxative—e.g., bisacodyl (Dulcolax)—the afternoon before the examination, liquid meal in the evening
- Fasting, nothing p.o. on the day of examination
- Patient should have a full bladder for the examination

Materials

- Plastic tube with small metal tip
- Guide wire
- Mucosal anesthetic (e. g., Xylocaine gel) or spray for oral intubation
- Two catheter tip syringes
- Two vessels for contrast medium and methylcellulose
- Adapter for connecting syringe and tube
  or
- Pump and containers for the contrast medium and cellulose, with appropriate tubing
- Contrast and distension preparations (G. Antes method): 500 (to 900) mL diluted contrast medium (specific weight 1.2–1.3—e. g., Micropaque diluted 1 : 2 with water), 1500 (to 2000) mL methylcellulose (10 g dissolved in 0.2 L water heated to about 60 °C and mixed well, 1800 mL cold water added and mixed once more). Instillation temperature 18 °C (64.4 °F) (or body temperature)
- Image receiver system (e. g. films): three 24 × 30 cm (10 × 12"), two 35 × 35 cm (14 × 14")
- Image receiver dosage (sensitivity class): ≤ 5 µGy (SC 400)
- Object–detector distance: as small as possible
- Exposure: 110–130 kV, automatic, center cell
- Focal spot nominal value: ≤ 1.3

Examination Technique

- Preliminary fluoroscopic check (for residual contrast, free air, bowel-gas pattern)
- After local anesthesia of the nasopharynx, the tube, with stiff guide wire, is inserted through the nose, with the patient erect
- The tube is then advanced, and the patient is put into a horizontal position (first on the right side to pass through the pylorus, then on the left side for passage through the duodenal loop, tip of the tube flexible)
- Distal portion of the tube is advanced beyond the ligament of Treitz (to prevent reflux)
- Contrast instillation, first under fluoro, of about 300 mL at a flow rate of 80 mL/min

1st film: single contrast view of the jejunum
- 24 × 30 cm (10 × 12"), landscape or portrait
- Immediate and quick instillation of methylcellulose at a flow rate of about 100–200 mL/min; total volume mostly 500–1500 mL, depending on the length of the intestine

2nd–3rd film: jejunum and ileum, double contrast views, cecum
– 24×30 cm (10×12"), divided as necessary for good demonstration, compression spots if needed

4th–5th film: jejunum and ileum, double-contrast views (survey films, depending on findings; either oblique or in prone and supine positions)
– 35×35 cm (14×17")

Follow-up

– Tube removal

❗ Tips & Tricks

– When in doubt, use less contrast and more methylcellulose. If this results in poor contrast visualization of the proximal jejunum because of too much dilution, 50–100 mL barium can be added in between the methylcellulose injections

Patient Preparation

- Two days before the examination, begin dietary and laxative—e. g., senna (X-Prep), bisacodyl (Dulcolax); preparations as per instruction

Materials and Radiographic Technique

- Contrast medium (about 50 g barium sulfate/100 mL approx. 1.0–1.5 L, warmed up)
- Disposable enema bag with hose, enema tip (olive), and Y-connection with rubber ball for air insufflation (e. g., pneumocolon)
- Contrast pump with connections and colon tube (additional pressure gauge and connections)
- Image receiver system (e. g. film sizes): four 24×30 cm (10×12"), two 35×35 cm (14×14")
- Image receiver dosage (sensitivity class): ≤5 μGy (SC 400)
- Object–detector distance: as small as possible
- Exposure: ≥110 kV, automatic, center cell
- Focal spot nominal value: ≤1.3
- Bucky: r 8
- Starting position of the fluoro unit: horizontal

Examination Technique

- Preliminary fluoroscopic check (for residual contrast, calcifications, free air?)
- Brief rectal examination (stenosis, tumor; blood or feces on glove?)
- Insert rectal tip
- Patient lies on the left side
- Instillation of the contrast medium under fluoroscopic control and under increased pressure if necessary (e. g., contrast pump)
- Retrograde flow of the contrast medium past the splenic flexure into the beginning or distal portion of the transverse colon
- The contrast is then advanced further just beyond the right flexure by turning the patient on the right side or by air insufflation
- Have the patient get up and evacuate the contrast material (either into the enema bag, or patient is sent to the toilet)
- Next, air insufflation with the patient lying on the left side (pump with controlled pressure if needed), under fluoroscopic control until the bowel segments of interest are distended

1st film: sigmoid rotated free of superimposed bowel loops

- Positioning under fluoroscopy (supine position, either left or right side slightly turned up)
- 24×30 cm (10×12"), landscape, undivided

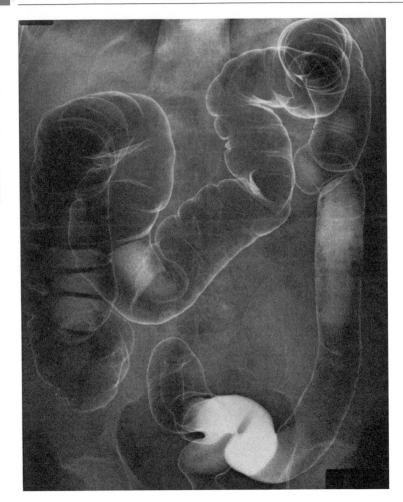

2nd film:
- 24×30 cm (10×12"), landscape, divided in two
  1st exposure: double-contrast view of the lateral rectum (shows the anterior margin of the sacrum, femoral heads are superimposed on each other), left lateral position
  2nd exposure: double-contrast view of the AP rectum, supine position (or prone, with head lowered)

3rd film: AP view of the transverse colon (cecum may also be clearly projected)
- Supine position
- 35×35 cm (14×14"), undivided

4th film: left colonic (splenic) flexure
- Positioned fluoroscopically, erect, usually LAO
- 24×30 cm (10×12"), portrait, undivided

5th film: right colonic (hepatic) flexure
- Positioned fluoroscopically, erect, usually RAO
- 24×30 cm (10×12"), portrait, undivided

6th film: survey film
- Erect AP
- 35×35 cm (14×14"), undivided

Variations

Variation in examining technique: hypotonic study of the colon
Materials (in addition to the above)
- 18-gauge needle
- 2 mL syringe with 2 mL Buscopan (20 mg) (caution: glaucoma and tachycardia)
  or
- Insulin syringe with 15 graduations = 0.4 mg glucagon
- Skin preparation, sponges, tourniquet
- Injection of Buscopan (20 mg) (or glucagon) prior to the instillation (or when needed)

Variation in radiographic technique: Bucky table method (Welin technique)
- Films: six 24×30 cm (10×12"), five 30×40 cm (12×16")
- Sensitivity class: 400
- SID: 115 cm (40")
- Bucky: yes (under the table, r 8)
- Focal spot size (large (focal spot nominal value: ≤ 1.3)
- Exposure: ≥ 100 kV, automatic, cell depending on position (middle or both lateral cells)

Other materials and technique as above
1st film: double-contrast view of the rectum, PA
- Prone position
- 24×30 cm (10×12"), undivided

2nd and 3rd films: rectum, raised right or left
- Prone position, raised about 30–40°
- 24×30 cm (10×12"), undivided

4th film: rectum, lateral projection
- Left lateral position
- 24×30 cm (10×12"), portrait, undivided

5th and 6th films: supine films of the abdomen, right and left oblique views
- Supine position, 30–45° rotation, centered at the umbilicus
- 30×40 cm (12×16"), undivided

7th film: recumbent film of the abdomen, horizontal projection
- Left lateral position, centered at the umbilicus
- 30×40 cm (12×16"), undivided

8th film: recumbent film of the abdomen, horizontal projection
- Right lateral position, centered at the umbilicus
- 30×40 cm (12×16"), undivided

9th film: erect film of the abdomen
- Centered at the umbilicus
- 30×40 cm (12×16"), undivided

10th film: erect film of the abdomen (for the right colonic flexure)
- 45° RAO, centered 2 FB above the umbilicus, right upper abdomen
- 24×30 cm (10×12"), undivided

11th film: erect film of the abdomen (for the left colonic flexure)
- 45° LAO, centered 4 FB above the umbilicus, left upper abdomen
- 24×30 cm (10×12"), undivided

Complications and How to Manage Them

- Rectal perforation: special caution is required when starting to instill contrast and air
- Pain during air insufflation: may be due to overdistension of a bowel segment. It may help to change the patient's position (turning the more proximal, undistended bowel loop upward)
- If the bowel loops do not open out: inject Buscopan (see *Variations*)

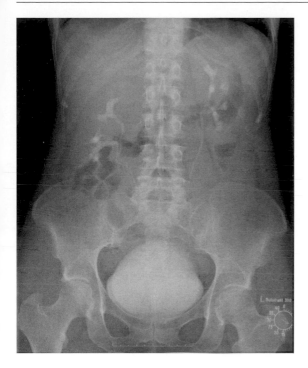

■ **Patient Preparation**

– Fasting for 3 h before the examination
– Laxatives and bowel cleansing the day before
– Creatinine less than 3 mg/dL (with larger doses of contrast medium up to 6 mg/dL)

Materials and Radiographic Technique

–   Contrast medium (dosage: adults 1 mL/kg body weight; children up to age 1, 3 mL/kg body weight [20 mL maximum, 12 mL minimum dose]; up to age 2, 2.5 mL/kg body weight [20 mL maximum dose]; up to age 3, 1.5 mL/kg body weight [25 mL maximum dose]; mostly 60%)
–   Butterfly or indwelling catheter (21 or 18 gauge)
–   Image receiver system (e.g. film sizes): two 35 × 35 cm (14 × 14") (in ideal conditions)
–   Image receiver dosage (sensitivity class): ≤ 5 μGy (SC 400)
–   SID: 115 cm (40")
–   Bucky: yes (under the table, r 12 [8])
–   Focal spot size: large (focal spot nominal value ≤ 1.3)
–   Exposure: 70–90 kV, automatic, both outer cells

Examination Technique

1st film: 35 × 43 cm (14 × 17"), portrait, undivided
–   Preliminary film
–   Supine position, lower film edge = upper border of the pubic symphysis
–   Additional oblique or preliminary tomographic view
–   Injection of the contrast medium
2nd film: 35 × 43 cm (14 × 17"), portrait, undivided
–   14 min after the injection
–   Supine position, lower film edge = upper border of the pubic symphysis
–   Additional views as needed
Zonography
–   24 × 30 cm (10 × 12"), undivided
–   Linear blurring, 8° exposure angle
–   Depth of slices about 8–9 cm, exposure time about 2 s
–   Supine position, centering over the kidney region (upper cassette border at about the level of the xiphoid process)
If *tomographic views* are required
–   Three 24 × 30 cm (10 × 12"), portrait, undivided
–   Linear blurring, 30° amplitude
–   Tomographic cuts at 1-cm intervals
–   Centering over the kidneys
–   Tomographic cuts at 9, 10, 11 cm (normal patients)

Lateral oblique views if needed
Compression films (for better filling of the renal pelves)
(Caution is required with compression if there is any obstruction of urinary drainage or infection)
– Either application of compression belt or patient in prone position, film taken after 15 minutes
Either
– 24×30 cm (10×12"), landscape, undivided
– Supine position, centering over the kidneys
or
– 35×43 cm (14×17"), portrait, undivided
– Supine position (remove compression belt)
– Lower film edge = upper border of the symphysis
Bladder films
1st film: full bladder
– 24×30 cm (10×12"), portrait, undivided
– Lower film edge = 2 cm below upper border of the symphysis
2nd film: bladder after voiding
– 18×24 cm (8×10"), landscape, undivided
– Lower film edge = 2 cm below upper border of the symphysis
All films are taken in expiration and with breath-holding
Delayed films for follow-up (e.g., nonfunctioning kidney, obstruction): 30 min, 1, 2, 12, 24 h post injection

Variations

(As part of excretory function studies)
– Erect urogram AP or in lateral projection, at rest, and attempting to strain and bear down
– Early urogram in AP supine position in case of suspected renal artery stenosis
– Breathing urogram to evaluate inflammatory fixation of the kidney in AP projection with long exposure time and low mA
– Oblique views for question of ureteral calculus: opposite side turned up 45° (if calculus is suspected behind the bladder, same side oblique 45°)

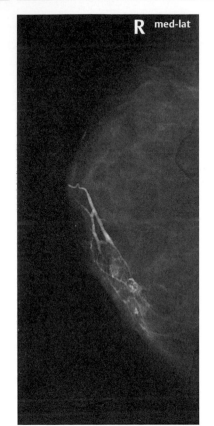

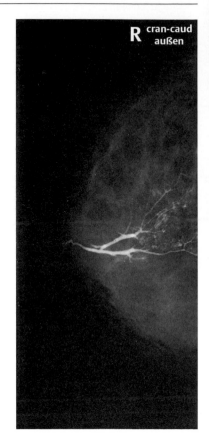

▨ Patient Preparation

– Mammography in two planes

Materials (sterile)

– Plastic tube with attached blunt cannula with end hole (e. g., galactography set) or dilators sizes 7, 8 and blunt cannulas sizes 7, 8
– 2 mL syringe with contrast medium (50 %)
– Spray dressing
– Sterile towels, sponges, gloves
– Skin disinfectant

Examination Technique

– After cleaning the nipple, controlled compression of the breast until the opening of the secreting mammary duct becomes moist
– Smear of mamillary secretion for cytological examination
– Dilation of the duct, if necessary
– Insertion of the blunt cannula
– Lifting and compression of the nipple
– Injection of 0.5–2.0 mL contrast medium (no air!)
– Note any sensations of discomfort for the patient (feelings of tenseness, aching pain)
– After removal of the cannula, closure of the mammary duct by compression (and spray dressing if necessary)

Radiographs

Mammography in two planes with moderate compression to prevent leaking of the contrast medium

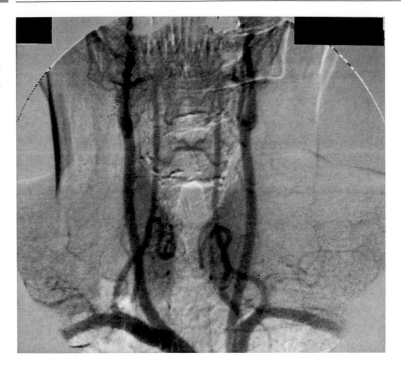

Radiographic Protocol

- At least two images per second
- After breathing instructions, contrast medium is injected, breath is held in mid-respiration
- Masks are prepared at the same time
- Wait for the end of the venous phase (series takes about 12 s, extended to 20 s if there is arterial occlusion—e. g., subclavian steal syndrome)
- Series is terminated

1st series
- Survey film of the aortic arch (30–45° LAO, 10–20° craniocaudad tube angulation for origin of the great vessels)

2nd series
- Neck LAO, head turned left (with electronic image magnification)

3rd series
- Neck RAO, head turned right (with electronic image magnification)

4th series
- Neck AP, 30–40° craniocaudad tube angulation (with electronic magnification, cervicocranial vascular junction)

■ **Patient Preparation**

– Fasting for at least 3 h
– Patient information and consent discussion, inquiry about renal and thyroid function (creatinine?)
– Removal of jewelry, glasses, removable dentures

Equipment and Materials

DSA table (peripheral venous)
– Two large syringes (20 or 30 mL) with NaCl
– 2-mL syringe with 21-gauge needle for local anesthesia
– Sponges
– Skin disinfectant
– Tourniquet
– Sterile bandages
Catheters
– Indwelling or butterfly needles, 14- and 16-gauge
– High-pressure two-way stopcock
– High-pressure connection tube, with clamps to attach to the table

▲ **Positioning**

– Supine (arm may be laid on a rest if needed)

Technical Preparations

– Fill the injection syringe

Puncture

– After local anesthesia, needle puncture of the median cubital vein
– Connecting tube attached (make sure there is no air in the tubing)
– Test injection of saline under rapid flow
– Connection to the injector (connecting tube fastened and high-pressure two-way stopcock)
– Raise the arm above the head to straighten the inflow tract

Injection Parameters

– About 50 mL nonionic contrast medium (350–370 mg iodine/mL contrast)
– Injection speed:
   about 14–16 mL/s with 16-gauge needle
   18–22 mL/s with 14-gauge needle

Follow-up

– Check for reaction to the contrast medium
– Pressure dressing

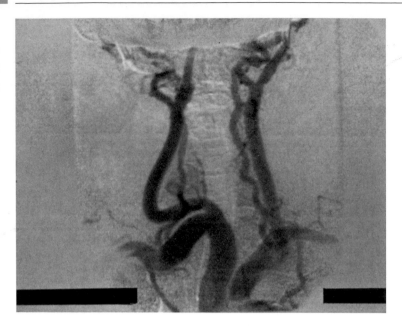

Patient Preparation

- Fasting for at least 3 h
- Clotting tests (Quick test, PT, PTT), creatinine
- Chest X-ray
- Patient information and consent discussion, inquiry about renal and thyroid function

Equipment and Materials

DSA table (central venous, sterile)
- Basin with NaCl and heparin (200 IU/10 mL)
- Two large syringes (20 or 30 mL) for NaCl
- One large syringe (20–30 mL, Luer) for the contrast medium
- 10-mL syringe with 21-gauge (green) needle for local anesthesia (or 2-mL syringe with 18-gauge needle for venous puncture in the arm)
- Puncture needle (e.g., 18 gauge for 0.38" or 19 gauge for 0.35" guide wire)
- Scalpel
- High-pressure two-way stopcock
- Sterile sponges (e.g., 10 small, 10 large)

- Sterile towels, gloves
- Contrast medium, local anesthetic
- Skin disinfectant (e.g., Betadine)
- Disposable razor for femoral vein

Catheters
- 5-French pigtail catheter, length 65 cm (for femoral vein puncture) or 90 cm (for arm vein puncture)
- Puncture needle (e.g., 18 gauge for 0.38" or 19 gauge for 0.35" guide wire)
- J-guide (e.g., 0.38" or 0.35", 150 cm long)

▲ Positioning
- Supine (arm may be laid on a rest if needed)

Technical Preparations
- Syringe filled for injection, free of air

Puncture
- Femoral or median cubital vein punctured after local anesthesia and skin incision
- The catheter is advanced along the inserted guide wire into the superior vena cava just above the right atrium
- Trial injection to check position
- Connection to the injector (after the air is out)

Injection Parameters
- About 30–50 mL nonionic contrast medium (300–330 mg iodine/mL contrast)
- Injection speed: 15–20 mL/s

Radiographic Protocol
- At least two images per second
- After breathing instructions, injection of the contrast medium, respiration suspended in expiration
- At the same time, a mask is prepared
- Wait for the venous phase (series takes about 12 s, or as long as 20 s if there is arterial occlusion (e.g., in subclavian steal syndrome)
- Terminate the series

1st series
- Survey films of the aortic arch (30–45° LAO, 10–20° craniocaudad tube angulation for origin of the great vessels)

2nd series
– Neck LAO, head turned left (with electronic image magnification)
3rd series
– Neck RAO, head turned right (with electronic image magnification)
4th series
– Neck AP, 30–40° craniocaudad tube angulation (with electronic image magnification, cervicocranial vascular junction)

Follow-up

– Check for reaction to the contrast medium
– About 5 min compression (5–10 for the femoral vein)
– Pressure dressing applied to the puncture site
– Recheck about 30 min before discharge

Patient Preparation

– Fasting for 3 h
– Clotting tests (Quick test, PTT, thrombocytes)
– Chest X-ray in two projections
– Patient information and consent discussion, inquiry about renal and thyroid function
– Jewelry, glasses, and dentures should be removed

Equipment and Materials

Angio table (sterile)
– Basin with NaCl and heparin (200 IU/100 mL)
– Two large syringes (20 or 30 mL)
– One large contrast syringe (Luer, 20 mL)
– 10-mL syringe with 21- and 23-gauge needles for local anesthesia
– Sponges (e.g., 10 small, 10 large)
– Scalpel
– Puncture needle (e.g., 18-gauge for 0.38" or 19-gauge for 0.35" guide wire)
– High-pressure two-way stopcock
– Sterile towels
– Sterile coat, gloves
– Disposable razor
– Skin disinfectant (e.g., Betadine)
  Contrast medium, local anesthetic

Catheters
– 5-French pigtail catheter (100 cm)
– J-guide with soft tip (e.g., 0.38" or 0.35", 120–150 cm long)

▲ **Positioning**

– Supine position
– Shaving of the inguinal areas
– Skin disinfection
– Cover with sterile towels

Technical Preparations

– Syringe filled for injection, free of air

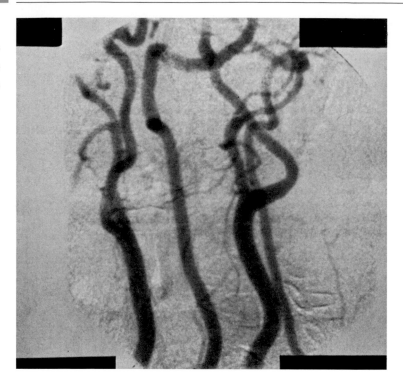

Puncture (Seldinger Technique)

- Femoral artery punctured after local anesthesia (pulsating jet of blood)
- Insertion of the J-guide
- Puncture needle is removed
- Catheter is inserted and advanced forward along the guide
- The guide is then removed
- Catheter placed at the origin of the ascending aorta (about 2 cm distal to the aortic valve)
- Preliminary aspiration of blood, saline injection (free runoff), test dose of contrast to check position
- Connection to the injector

Injection Parameters

- 30–40 mL nonionic contrast medium (300–330 mg iodine/mL)
- Injection speed 10–15 mL/s
- No injection delay

Radiographic Protocol

- Four images per second
- Injection after masks have been prepared
- Respiration suspended in expiration

1st series

- Survey films of the aortic arch (30–45° LAO; tip: catheter turned up under fluoroscopy)
- 10–20° craniocaudad tube angulation

2nd series

- Supine position, neck LAO (magnifying technique)
- Head turned left (about 30–40° LAO)

3rd series

- Supine position, neck RAO (magnifying technique)
- Head turned right (about 30–45° RAO)

4th series (optional)

- Supine position, neck AP (magnifying technique)
- 30° craniocaudad tube angulation

Follow-up

- Check for reaction to the contrast medium
- Compression of the puncture site for about 10 min
- Pressure dressing
- Bed rest (12–24 h)

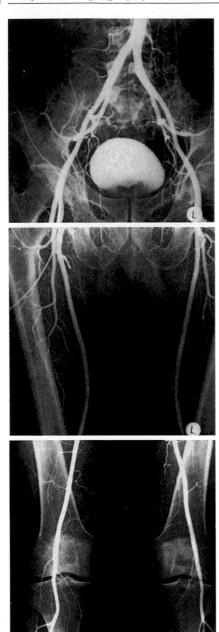

■ **Patient Preparation**

- Fasting for 3–6 h
- Clotting tests (e.g., Quick test over 50%, PT, PTT, thrombocytes)
- Creatinine
- Patient information and consent discussion, inquiry about thyroid disease

Equipment, Materials, and Radiographic Technique

Angio table (sterile)

- Basin with NaCl and heparin (200 IU/100 mL)
- Two large syringes (20 or 30 mL) for NaCl
- One large contrast syringe (Luer, 20 mL)
- 10-mL syringe with 21- and 23-gauge needles for local anesthesia
- Sponges (e.g., 10 small, 10 large)
- Scalpel
- Puncture needle (e.g., 19-gauge for 0.35" guide wire)
- Two-way stopcock
- Sterile towels
- Sterile coat, gloves
- Skin disinfectant, contrast medium, local anesthetic
- Disposable razor
- Films: load 10 cassette films
- Tube settings: about 66 kV (64 mAs [trial], negative step-down: 5, 15, 20, 25 kV)

Catheters

- 5-French pigtail catheter (65 cm)
- J-guide with soft tip (e.g., 0.35", 120–150 cm long)

▲ **Positioning**

- Supine position
- Shaving of the inguinal areas
- Skin disinfection
- Cover with sterile towels

Technical Preparations

- Take a survey film (central ray about 7 cm above the umbilicus to include the renal vessels, or 7 cm below umbilicus without renal vessels)
- Syringe filled for injection

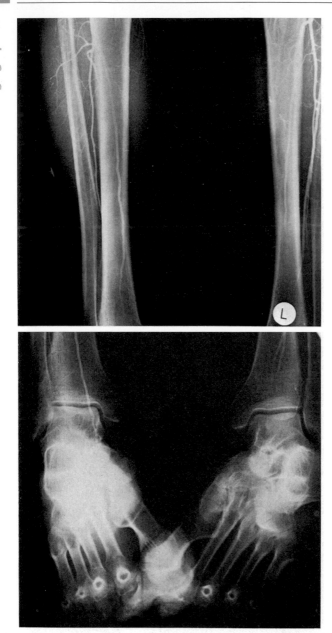

Puncture (Seldinger Technique)

- Femoral artery punctured after local anesthesia (pulsating jet of blood)
- Insertion of the J-guide
- The puncture needle is withdrawn, a dilator may be put in place
- Catheter, with open stopcock, is inserted and advanced forward along the guide
- The guide is removed, catheter flushed with NaCl, stopcock closed
- Catheter placed approx. 2 cm above the bifurcation, at about the level of L4 or at the renal artery level at L1–L2
- Test aspiration of blood, injection of NaCl (free runoff?)
- Catheter position checked with a test dose of the contrast medium
- Connection to the injector

Injection Parameters

- About 80 mL of nonionic contrast medium
- Injection speed and delay depending on the vascular situation or the flow-test injection, or on the walking distance
- Walking distance more than 200 m: flow = 11 mL/s, 3-s delay
- Walking distance about 100 m: flow 10 mL/s, 5-s delay
- Walking distance 20–50 m: flow 8 mL/s, 7–8-s delay

Radiographic Protocol

- Four table shifts = five filming stations
- At each station, one image per second twice
- Legs slightly rotated internally (with genu varum knee supported to compensate)
- Abdominal and pelvic levels in expiratory suspended respiration

Follow-up

- Check for reaction to the contrast medium
- 10 min compression of the puncture site
- Pressure dressing
- At least 24 h bed rest

! Tips & Tricks

- For patients less than 1.60 m (5½ feet) tall, only three table shifts = four filming stations = eight cassette films are needed

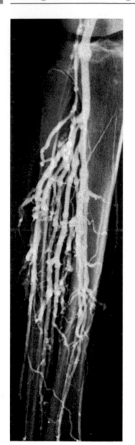
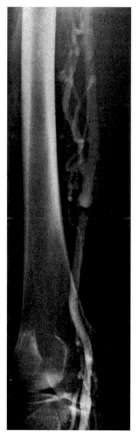
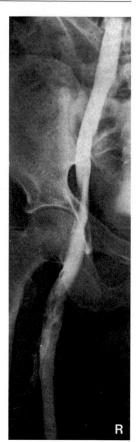

Patient Preparation

- Fasting for 3 h
- Patient information and consent discussion, inquiry about renal and thyroid function

Materials

- Butterfly needle (19–21 gauge) or Intracath in case of thrombolytic therapy
- One 20-mL syringe with 0.9% saline
- Three 20-mL syringes (or one 50-mL syringe) for contrast medium

- Tourniquet for application above the ankle
- A second tourniquet for application around the distal thigh
- Sponges, adhesive bandages, skin disinfectant
- Contrast medium
- Restraining belt
- Measuring rod
- Films: two 35×35 cm (14×14"), and two 10×20 cm (10×12") held ready

Examination Technique

- Application of a tourniquet above the ankle, puncture of a superficial vein in the dorsum of the foot with a butterfly needle after the air has been let out
- Puncture as distal as possible (mostly dorsal vein of the great toe)
- About 45° table tilt with the patient supine
- So-called "hanging position" with handles for support, or patient stands on one leg on a wooden block
- Attach measuring rod
- Manual injection of the contrast medium (40–60 mL)

1st film: 35×35 cm (14×14"), divided in three

- 1st exposure: lower leg in 30° internal rotation
- 2nd exposure: lower leg lateral (in maximal external rotation)
- 3rd exposure: knee region, including distal and midthigh (lateral, have patient strain: small saphenous vein)
- Ask patient to continue to strain, in order to get good filling for the runoff phase = 4th exposure
- Patient is placed in horizontal position under fluoroscopy, the leg is elevated, calf compressed (caution: possible thrombosis)

2nd film: 35×35 cm (14×14"), divided in three

- 4th exposure: middle and upper thigh (have patient strain)
- If the valves of the great saphenous vein are competent, continue with:
- 5th exposure: inguinal and iliac region
- 6th exposure: drainage into the inferior vena cava or delayed film of the lower leg in internal rotation

Follow-up

- Elevate and massage the leg
- Remove the needle, apply dressing, have patient walk up stairs
- Wrap the legs of bedridden patients

Variations

Variation in examination technique

In case of insufficiency of the great saphenous vein, the sequence of the second film is changed:

- 4th exposure: proximal thigh and inguinal region (demonstrating the drainage into the external and common iliac veins, and insufficiency of the valve
- 5th exposure: proximal and midportions of the insufficient great saphenous vein
- 6th exposure: distal insufficiency point of the great saphenous vein

! Tips & Tricks

- If not all veins of the lower leg fill right at the beginning, change the exposure sequence of the first film: 35×35 cm (14×14"), divided in three
  1st exposure: lateral knee and distal thigh
  2nd exposure: lateral lower leg
  3rd exposure: lower leg in 30° internal rotation
- If filling is still inadequate, squeeze the contrast material manually from the forefoot
- If filling is still incomplete, second injection after putting a second tourniquet around the distal thigh

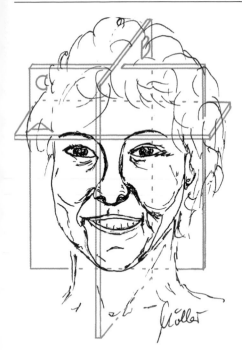

A = axial (horizontal) plane
B = sagittal plane
C = coronal (frontal) plane

Computed Tomography

Patient Preparation

- Fasting for 3 h if possible (due to contrast administration)
- Contrast administration if needed
- Laboratory values (creatinine, baseline thyroid-stimulating hormone), allergy history, inquiry regarding renal and thyroid function

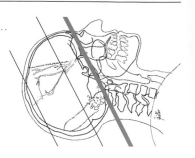

Materials

- 1 butterfly catheter (16 or 18 gauge) or 21-gauge (green) or 1-gauge (yellow) needle
- 1 (or 2) large 50-mL syringe (50–100 mL), filled with contrast medium (approximately 300 mg iodine/mL)
- Pressure dressing, swabs, skin disinfectant, adhesive bandages

▲ Positioning

- Supine, arms along the sides of the body
- Head positioned symmetrically, chin raised, head immobilized in head holder

Parameters

- Scan range start–end: 1st set of scans: foramen magnum—superior edge of petrous bone; 2nd set of scans: superior edge of petrous bone—roof of skull
- Breathing: shallow breathing
- Digital scout view: lateral (256 mm)
- Scanning unit tilt: parallel to the canthomeatal line
- Scan direction: caudocranial
- Reconstruction: soft-tissue filter (or in cases of fracture or metastasis: bone filter)

Documentation

- Soft-tissue window
- Posterior fossa: Window level (WL): 40–50 HU; window width (WW): 120–160 HU
- Rest of the neurocranium: WL 35–40 HU; ww 70–100 HU
- Bone window: WL 400–400 HU; ww approximately 2000 HU

▌ Tips & Tricks

- If the patient is unable to tilt the head back when coronal imaging is planned (e. g., sella, orbits): use axial slice technique with a 2-mm slice thickness and slice interval, or 1-mm slice thickness and pitch 1.0 (spiral). This is followed by secondary reconstruction.

– When there are dental fillings (causing artifacts), either tilt the gantry far enough for the fillings to be outside the slice level (semicoronal) or use the axial technique.
– Important: select the gantry tilt in such a way that the orbits are not in the radiation field.

Type/ orientation		Collimation (para-meters)	Speed	Pitch factor	Slice thick-ness	Scanning para-meters (kV)
For all						
1	Topo, lateral (256 mm)	1–3 mm				110–130
1-line						
2	Skull base, axial	4×1–2 mm	2–3	0.5–0.75	4 mm	120–140
3	Cerebrum, axial	4×2–4 mm	5–8	0.5–0.75	5–8 mm	120–140
2-line						
2	Skull base, axial	[2×]1–1.5 mm	2–3	1	3–4 mm	120–140
3	Cerebrum, axial	[2×]2–4 mm	5–8	1	5–8 mm	120–140
6-line						
2	Skull base, axial	[6×]1 mm	2–3	1	3–4 mm	120–140
3	Cerebrum, axial	[6×]2 mm	5–8	1	5–6 mm	120–140
16-line						
2	Skull base, axial	[16×]0.6–0.75 mm	5.3–7	0.5–0.6	3–4 mm	120–140
3	Cerebrum, axial	[16×]1.2–1.5 mm	10.6–14	0.55	5–6 mm	120–140
64-line						
2 (+3)	Skull base (+ Cerebrum), axial	[64×]0.6 mm	5.4	0.9	4–5 mm	120–140
4	Post contrast	Amount: 50–60 mL		Flow: 1–2 mL/s		Delay: 60–120 s

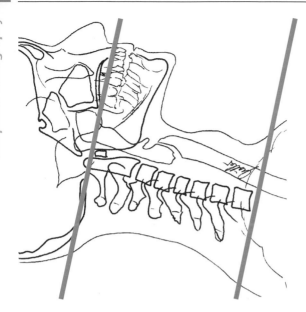

—— Slice boundaries for CT of the neck

Patient Preparation
- Fasting for 3 h (due to contrast administration)
- Remove dentures
- Laboratory values (creatinine, baseline thyroid-stimulating hormone), allergy history, inquiry regarding renal and thyroid function, medication history

Materials
Contrast administration is needed if soft tissues in the neck are being investigated.
- 1 indwelling or butterfly catheter (16- or 18-gauge)
- Injector with 100 mL contrast (approximately 300 mg iodine/mL)
- Pressure dressing, swabs, skin disinfectant, adhesive bandages

Positioning
- Supine, neck slightly stretched out

- Arms along the sides of the body, shoulders should be pulled down if appropriate (e. g., with aids: holding a rope that passes round the feet will pull the wrists downward)
- Head immobilized

Parameters

Spiral CT

- Scan range start: adjust the base of the skull (e. g., hard palate–back of the head) to the issue being investigated (e. g., floor of the mouth or thyroid gland)
- Scan range end: e. g., aortic arch (adjust to issue being investigated)
- Breathing: breath held, no swallowing
- Digital scout view: lateral (256 mm) or AP (256 mm or 512 mm)
- Scanning unit tilt: 0–20°
- Magnification: floor of the mouth or neck should fill the image as much as possible
- Scan direction: caudocranial
- Documentation, soft-tissue window:
  WL: 40–60 HU
  WW: 200–400 HU
- Reconstruction: Soft-tissue filter (core), bone filter if appropriate (e. g., when investigating fractures or tumor)

Type/ orientation	Collima-tion (para-meters)	Speed	Pitch factor	Slice thickness	Scanning para-meters (kV)
For all					
1 Topo AP (cor 512 mm) or lateral 256 mm	1–3 mm				110–130
Contrast medium application	Amount: 100–120 mL		Flow: 1.5–3 mL/s		Delay: 40–60 s (or 15–25 s = arterial)
Postcontrast:					
1-line					
2 Neck spiral, axial	3 / 5 mm	5 / 8	1.5–1.7	3–5 mm	120–140
2-line					
2 Neck spiral, axial	[2×] 2.5 (1.5) mm	5 (6)	1 (2)	5 (2) mm	120–130
6-line					
2 Neck spiral, axial	[6×] 2 mm	5–10	0.85	5 (1.25) mm	120–130
16-line					
2 Neck spiral, axial	[16×] 1.5–2 mm	10–36	0.85–1.5	3–5 mm	120–130
64-line					
2 Neck spiral, axial	[64×] 0.6 mm	17.3	0.9–1.2	5 (1.5) mm	120–130
Alternative two-stage application of contrast medium:					
2 Neck spiral, axial	Amount: 50 mL		Flow: 2 mL/s		Delay: 40 s
3 Neck spiral, axial, late image 180 s after con-trast injection, otherwise as for 2nd spiral	Amount: 50 mL		Flow: 1 mL/s		Delay: 40 s

Variation

For functional examinations in the larynx, a thin-slice technique (see above) over the larynx can be used during "e"-phonation (the patient voices the vowel "e" loud and long; this can be practiced with the patient beforehand, and the length of the slice can be adjusted to the patient's ability to hold the "e").

! Tips & Tricks

- The shoulder girdle should be pulled downward as much as possible (the patient can hold the ends of a rope with both hands—e.g., using loops at the top—and the middle of the rope can be passed round the feet so that the shoulders are pulled downward when the legs are stretched out)
- The lateral boundaries should not be selected too narrowly (to allow assessment of the transitions to the floor of the mouth and to the chest)
- The reconstruction increment for coronal and sagittal reconstructions should be approximately 70% of the reconstructed slice thickness
- Sagittal reconstructions should always be used the when clinical issue involves bone changes
- If pathology in the floor of the mouth, parotid, or thyroid is being investigated, the collimation and reconstructed slice thickness should be less than 5 mm

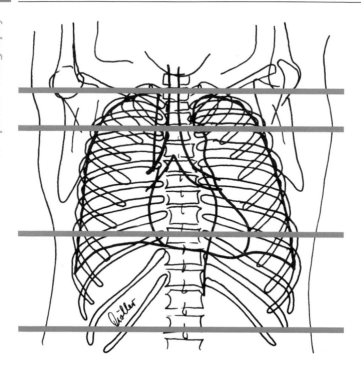

—— Slice boundaries for a normal chest examination
—— Slice boundaries for pulmonary embolism for 1–2-slice imaging

Patient Preparation

- Fasting for 3 h if possible (due to contrast administration)
- Chest radiograph at two levels
- Laboratory values (creatinine, baseline thyroid-stimulating hormone), allergy history, inquiry regarding renal and thyroid function, medication history

Materials

- 1 indwelling or butterfly catheter (16- or 18-gauge)
- 100 mL contrast (fill an injection syringe) or two 50-mL syringes filled with contrast (approximately 300 mg iodine/mL)
- Pressure dressing, swabs, skin disinfectant, adhesive bandages

▲ **Positioning**

– Supine, with the lower legs cushioned
– Arms folded behind the head

Parameters

– Scan range start: apex of the lungs
– Scan range end: lowest border of the dorsal recess (as far as about the middle of the renal shadow if there is a suspicion of tumor)
– Breathing: breath held in inspiration
– Scan direction: craniocaudal
– Reconstruction: soft-tissue filter and lung filter (core)
– Documentation
  Soft-tissue window:
  WL: 40–60 HU
  WW: 300–400 HU
  Lung window (identical for standard and high resolution):
  WL: –400 to –500 HU
  WW: 1500–2000 HU

Type/ orientation	Collimation (parameters)	Speed	Pitch factor	Slice thick- ness	Scanning param- eters (kV)
For all					
1 Scout view AP (lateral)	1–3 mm				100–130
Contrast medium application	Amount: 100–120 mL		Flow: 1.5–3 mL/s		Delay: 50–60 s
Postcontrast:					
1-line					
2 Chest spiral, axial, immediately after contrast (red lines)	5 mm	7.5	1.5–1.7	5 mm	130–140
Plus:					
3 Chest spiral from the lower end of the 1st spiral (lower red line) to the lower edge of the costodiaphragmatic recess (green line)	5 mm	7.5	1.5–1.7	5 mm	130–140
4 Chest spiral from the upper end of the 1st spiral (upper red line) to the apex of the chest (green line)	5 mm	7.5	1.5–1.7	5 mm	130–140
2-line					
2 Chest spiral, axial	[2×] 4 mm	16	2	5 mm	120–130
6-line					
2 Chest spiral, axial	[6×] 1.5–2 mm	9–18	1.5	4–5 mm	120–130
16-line					
2 Chest spiral, axial	[16×] 1.5–2 mm	9–18	1.0–1.5	3–5 mm	120–130
64-line					
2 Chest spiral, axial	[64×] 0.6 mm	26.9	1.4	3–5 mm	120–130

! **Tips & Tricks**

- A noncontrast series (for dose reduction) may occasionally be needed, depending on the issue being investigated (e. g., mediastinum always after contrast; exception: fresh bleeding following trauma)

- When there is a suspected tumor in the lung, at least both adrenal glands must be visible in the first examination (slice end at around the center of the kidney)

- If only one set of images is being sent by teleradiology, then the images using the lung filter (core) must be selected

- If there is a suspected pulmonary embolism: contrast amount 120–130 mL, delay 15–20 s (also for 1- or 2-slice), maximum slice thickness 5 mm

- The arm with the intravenous access should be stretched above the head and held and supported by the hand of the contralateral arm, which is folded behind the head (this provides stable and comfortable positioning and unobstructed contrast flow)

- If a device does not have a program for dosage modulation, weight-adjusted variation of the mAs is required (depending on the device type).

40–50 mAs	<60 kg patient weight
60 mAs	60–80 kg
80 mAs	80–100 kg
100–120 mAs	over 100 kg

- In patients with dyspnea or elderly patients and 1-slice or 2-slice imaging, two (or three) spirals are better:
  1. Spiral up to 2 cm below the carina of the trachea; then let the patient breathe briefly and start the second slice up to the dorsal recess
  2. Time contrast administration so that it is sufficient for the first spiral
  3. For patients with resting dyspnea, always run three spirals (as in 1-slice for pulmonary embolism; see above)

- Children:
  (a) Chest CT may be reduced to a slice thickness of 5 mm in children
  (b) Children should always be examined with a weight-adjusted dosage. Normally, the examination is carried out as low-dose CT (= 20 mAs). The pitch factor can be up to 2, depending on the issue being investigated

Computed Tomography

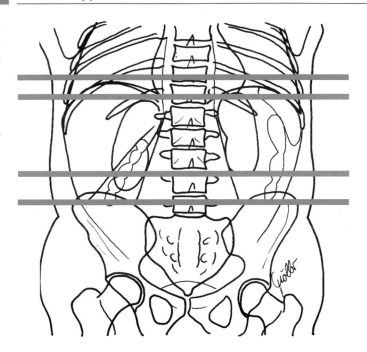

—— Slice boundaries for upper abdominal examination
—— Slice boundaries—e.g., for pancreatic thin-slice CT

Patient Preparation

– Fasting for 3 h (due to contrast administration)
– Laboratory values (creatinine, baseline thyroid-stimulating hormone), allergy history, inquiry regarding renal and thyroid function, medication history
– Approximately 30 min before the examination, fractionated oral administration of 500–600 mL of CT-suitable contrast. The last swallow should be taken just before the examination. The patient may be positioned on the right side for the topogram (to fill the duodenum when the pancreas is being investigated)

Computed Tomography

Materials

- 500–600 mL CT-suitable contrast
- Hyoscine butylbromide (Buscopan) or glucagon can be injected to reduce intestinal peristalsis, with a 2-mL syringe and an 18-gauge needle (if an indwelling or butterfly catheter has not been placed)

Intravenous contrast if needed:

- 1 indwelling or butterfly catheter (16- or 18-gauge)
- 100 mL contrast (fill an injection syringe) or two 50-mL syringes filled with contrast (approximately 300 mg iodine/mL)
- Pressure dressing, swabs, skin disinfectant, adhesive bandages

▲ Positioning

- Supine, with the lower legs cushioned
- Arms folded behind the head

Parameters

- Scan range start. Depending on the issue being investigated:
  Liver: 1st spiral, dome of diaphragm; 2nd spiral, dome of diaphragm
  Pancreas: 1st spiral, approximately T12; 2nd spiral, dome of diaphragm
  Kidneys: 1st spiral, upper pole of kidney; 2nd spiral, upper pole of kidney
- Scan range end: Depending on the issue being investigated:
  Liver: 1st spiral, tip of liver; 2nd spiral, tip of liver
  Pancreas: 1st spiral, lower edge of L2; 2nd spiral, tip of liver
  Kidneys: 1st spiral, pelvic inlet; 2nd spiral, lower edge of symphysis
- Breathing: breath held in inspiration
- Digital scout view: AP (512 mm)
- Scanning unit tilt: 0
- Scan direction: craniocaudal
- Documentation, soft-tissue window:
  WL: 40–60 HU
  WW: 200–500 HU

Type/ orientation		Collimation (parameters)	Speed	Pitch factor	Slice thickness	Scannin param- eters (k
For all						
1	Topo AP (cor) long (512 mm)	1–3 mm				100–13C
Contrast medium application		Amount: 100–120 mL		Flow: 2–3 mL/s		Delay: 15–30 s
Postcontrast:						
1-line						
2	Abdominal spiral, axial (over the organ)	(7) 8 mm	(7.5) 12.8	1.5–1.6	(7) 8 mm	120–13C
Immediately after:						
3	Upper abdominal spiral, axial	(7) 8 mm	(7.5) 12.8	1.5–1.6	(7) 8 mm	120–13C
2-line						
2	Organ spiral, axial	[2×] 4 mm	16	2	3.5–5 mm	110–130
3	Upper abdominal spiral, axial	[2×] 5 mm	15–20	1.5–2	5–8 mm	110–130
6-line						
2	Organ spiral, axial	[6×] 1 mm	9–10	1.25	1.25– 3 mm	120–130
3	Upper abdominal spiral, axial	[6×] 2 mm	9–10	1.25	5–6 mm	120–130
16-line						
2	Organ spiral, axial	[16×] 1 mm	16–24	1.0–1.5	1–3 mm	120–130
3	Upper abdominal spiral, axial	[16×] 1.5 mm	24–36	1.0–1.5	4–6 mm	120–130
64-line						
2	Organ spiral, axial	[64×] 0.6 mm	26.9	1.4	1–3 mm	120–130
3	Upper abdominal spiral, axial	[64×] 0.6 mm	26.9	1.4	4–6 mm	120–130
Non- contrast	For specific investigations (e. g., calculus), noncontrast imaging can be carried out before contrast administration either as an upper abdominal or abdominal study					

Variation

"Routine upper abdomen":

– Depending on the issue being investigated, often just a single upper abdominal spiral: scan start at dome of the diaphragm, scan end at around the center of the kidney, contrast delay 40–60 s, otherwise as (3) upper abdominal spiral

Three-phase upper abdominal CT (e.g., to investigate hepatic or pancreatic tumors). Following (1) the scout view and (2) the upper abdominal spiral twice in succession:

– (2) Organ (or upper abdomen) spiral, approx. 15–25 s delay (arterial phase)
– (3) Organ (or upper abdomen) spiral, approx. 30–40 s delay (portal venous phase)
– (4) Upper abdominal spiral, approx. 60–80 s delay (venous phase)

Depending on the device, the first two spirals can be carried out in fast mode. For timing, bolus tracking may be useful if available (region of interest in the proximal abdominal aorta, density value for resolution to 120 HU)

! Tips & Tricks

– A dilute barium solution (1–2%), water-soluble contrast containing iodine (2–4%), or simply water can be used as oral contrast media. For investigations of the liver, gallbladder, pancreas, stomach, and bowel, focal lesions in the kidney, and CT angiography, water is actually better
– Late imaging can be carried out if there is poor bowel contrast or after intravenous contrast injection—e.g., if there is a questionable renal or bladder process
– In spiral CT involving longer examination times, patients should be asked to hyperventilate before the spiral (caution is needed here in older patients)
– If there is known cardiac insufficiency, the delay can be extended
– If there are "poor" veins, reduce the flow (rule of thumb: flow –0.5 ml = delay + 10 s)
– If pancreatic changes are being investigated, two ampoules of intravenous Buscopan can be administered shortly before the examination

Caution:

– In patients with pheochromocytoma, intravenous contrast administration can trigger a hypertensive crisis
– If a possible intestinal stenosis is being investigated, only water or a water-soluble contrast medium should be used

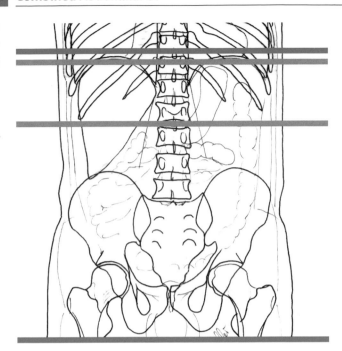

—— Slice boundaries for upper abdominal examination (e. g., pancreas)
—— Slice boundaries for abdominal examination

Patient Preparation

- Fasting for 3 h (due to contrast administration)
- Laboratory values (creatinine, baseline thyroid-stimulating hormone), allergy history, inquiry regarding renal and thyroid function, medication history
- Approximately 30 min before the examination, fractionated oral administration of 500 mL of CT-suitable contrast. The last swallow should be taken just before the examination. The patient may be positioned on the right side for the topogram (to fill the duodenum when the pancreas is being investigated)

Computed Tomography

Materials

- 100 mL CT-suitable contrast
- Rectal instillation of suitable contrast is possible (as a single enema =200 mL or approx. 200–500 mL in a disposable colon bag with inflow tube)
- Hyoscine butylbromide (Buscopan) or glucagon can be injected to reduce intestinal peristalsis, with a 2-mL syringe and an 18-gauge needle (if an indwelling or butterfly catheter has not been placed)

Intravenous contrast if needed:

- 1 indwelling or butterfly catheter (16- or 18-gauge)
  100 mL contrast (fill an injection syringe) or two 50 mL syringes filled with contrast (approximately 300 mg iodine/mL)
- Pressure dressing, swabs, skin disinfectant, adhesive bandages

▲ Positioning

- Supine, with the lower legs cushioned
- Arms folded behind the head

Parameters

- Scan range start:
  1st spiral (upper abdomen): depending on the issue being investigated
  (e.g., *pancreas:* upper edge of T12, *liver:* dome of the diaphragm
  2nd spiral, dome of the diaphragm
- Scan range end:
  1st spiral (upper abdomen), depending on the issue being investigated
  (e.g., *pancreas:* lower edge of L2, *liver:* tip of the liver usually at the level of the ala of the ilium
  2nd spiral, lower edge of ischium
- Breathing: breath held in inspiration
- Digital scout view: AP (512 mm)
- Scanning unit tilt: 0
- Scan direction: craniocaudal
- Documentation, soft-tissue window:
  WL: 40–60 HU
  WW: 200–500 HU

Type/ orientation		Collimation (parameters)	Speed	Pitch factor	Slice thickness	Scanning parameters (kV
For all						
1	Scout AP (cor) long (512 mm)	1–3 mm				100–130
Contrast medium application		Amount: 100–120 mL		Flow: 2–3 mL/s		Delay: 15–30 s
Postcontrast:						
1-line						
2	Abdominal spiral, axial (over the organ)	(7) 8 mm	(7.5) 12.8	1.5–1.6	(7) 8 mm	110–130
Immediately after:						
3	Upper abdominal spiral, axial	(7) 8 mm	(7.5) 12.8	1.5–1.6	(7) 8 mm	110–130
2-line						
2	Organ spiral, axial	[2×] 4 mm	16	2	3.5–5 mm	110–130
3	Upper abdominal spiral, axial	[2×] 5 mm	20	2	5–8 mm	110–130
6-line						
2	Upper abdominal spiral, axial	[6×] 1 mm	9	1.5	1.25–3 mm	120–130
3	Abdominal spiral, axial	[6×] 2 mm	10	0.85	5–6 mm	120–130
16-line						
2	Upper abdominal spiral, axial	[16×] 1.5–2 mm	9–18	1.0–1.5	1.25–3 mm	120–130
3	Abdominal spiral, axial	[16×] 1.5–2 mm	9–18	1.0–1.5	4–6 mm	120–130
64-line						
2	Upper abdominal spiral, axial	[64×] 0.6 mm	26.9	1.4	1–3 mm	120–130
3	Abdominal spiral, axial	[64×] 0.6 mm	26.9	1.4	4–6 mm	120–130
Noncontrast	For specific investigations (e.g., calcification, calculus), noncontrast imaging can be carried out before contrast administration either as an upper abdominal or abdominal study					

Variations

Three-phase upper abdominal CT (e.g., to investigate hepatic or pancreatic tumors). Following (1) the scout view and (2) the upper abdominal spiral twice in succession:

- (2) Upper abdominal spiral, approx. 15–25 s delay (arterial phase)
- (3) Upper abdominal spiral, approx. 30–40 s delay (portal venous phase)
- (4) Abdominal spiral, approx. 60–80 s delay (venous phase)

Depending on the device, fast mode can be used for the upper abdominal spirals. For timing, bolus tracking may be useful if available (region of interest in the proximal abdominal aorta)

! Tips & Tricks

- A dilute barium solution (1–2%), water-soluble contrast containing iodine (2–4%), or simply water can be used as oral contrast media. For investigations of the liver, gallbladder, pancreas, stomach, and bowel, focal lesions in the kidney, and CT angiography, water is actually better
- Negative contrast of the intestines is also possible (with instillation of cooking oil—e.g., for examinations of the colon)
- Late imaging can be carried out if there is poor bowel contrast or after intravenous contrast injection—e.g., if there is a questionable renal or bladder process
- In spiral CT involving longer examination times, patients should be asked to hyperventilate before the spiral (caution is needed here in older patients).
- If there is known cardiac insufficiency, the delay can be extended
- If there are "poor" veins, reduce the flow (rule of thumb: flow −0.5 mL = delay + 10 s)
- If pancreatic changes are being investigated, two ampoules of intravenous Buscopan can be administered shortly before the examination
- Caution:
- In patients with pheochromocytoma, intravenous contrast administration can trigger a hypertensive crisis
- If a possible intestinal stenosis is being investigated, only water or a water-soluble contrast medium should be used

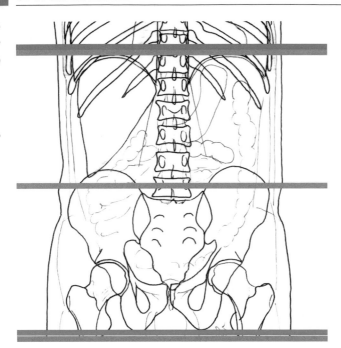

—— Slice boundaries for a normal abdominal examination
—— Slice boundaries for two-part procedure for 1-slice study (one pause for one breathing command)

Patient Preparation

- Fasting for 3 h (due to contrast administration)
- Approximately 60–90 min before the examination, fractionated oral administration of 1000 mL of CT-suitable contrast until just before the start of the examination (approx. 5 min before)
- A few more swallows of contrast should be taken just before the examination
- A vaginal tampon may be inserted if appropriate
- Rectal instillation of suitable contrast if appropriate
- Laboratory values (creatinine, baseline thyroid-stimulating hormone), allergy history, inquiry regarding renal and thyroid function, medication history

Computed Tomography

Materials

- Intravenous contrast if needed:
- 1 indwelling or butterfly catheter (16- or 18-gauge)
- 100 mL contrast (fill an injection syringe) or two 50-mL syringes filled with contrast (approximately 300 mg iodine/mL)
- Pressure dressing, swabs, skin disinfectant, adhesive bandages

▲ Positioning

- Supine, with the lower legs cushioned
- Arms folded behind the head

Parameters

- Scan range start: dome of the diaphragm
- Scan range end: at about the lower edge of ischium
- Breathing: breath held in inspiration
- Digital scout view: AP (512 mm)
- Scanning unit tilt: 0
- Scan direction: craniocaudal
- Documentation, soft-tissue window:
  WL: 40–60 HU
  WW: 200–500 HU

Type/ orientation		Collimation (parameters)	Speed	Pitch factor	Slice thickness	Scanning parameters (kV)
For all						
1	Scout AP (lat)	1–3 mm				100–130
Contrast medium application		Amount: 100–120 mL		Flow: 2–3 mL/s		Delay: 50–60 s
Postcontrast:						
1-line						
2	Abdominal spiral, axial	(7) 8 mm	(7.5) 12.8	1.5–1.6	(7) 8 mm	110–130
Depending on the device, two spiral sets may be needed (e.g., upper abdomen and pelvis) with a very short pause for one breathing command						
2-line						
2	Organ spiral, axial	[2×] 5 mm	20	2	5–8 mm	120–130
6-line						
2	Upper abdominal spiral, axial	[6×] 2 mm	10	0.85	5–6 mm	120–130
16-line						
2	Upper abdominal spiral, axial	[16×] 1.5–2 mm	24–36	1.0–1.5	5–6 mm	120–130
64-line						
2	Upper abdominal spiral, axial	[64×] 0.6 mm	26.9	1.4	5 mm	120–130

! Tips & Tricks

- A dilute barium solution (1–2%), water-soluble contrast containing iodine (2–4%), or simply water can be used as oral contrast media. For investigations of the liver, gallbladder, pancreas, stomach, and bowel, focal lesions in the kidney, and CT angiography, water is actually better
- Negative contrast of the intestines is also possible (with instillation of cooking oil—e. g., for examinations of the colon)
- Late imaging can be carried out if there is poor bowel contrast or after intravenous contrast injection—e. g., if there is a questionable renal or bladder process
- In spiral CT involving longer examination times, patients should be asked to hyperventilate before the spiral (caution is needed here in older patients).
- The reconstruction increment for coronal and sagittal reconstructions should be approximately 70% of the reconstructed slice thickness
- Noncontrast abdominal spirals are usually only need for investigating calcification (calculus), or when contrast is contraindicated

Caution:

- In patients with pheochromocytoma, intravenous contrast administration can trigger a hypertensive crisis
- If a possible intestinal stenosis is being investigated, only water or a water-soluble contrast medium should be used

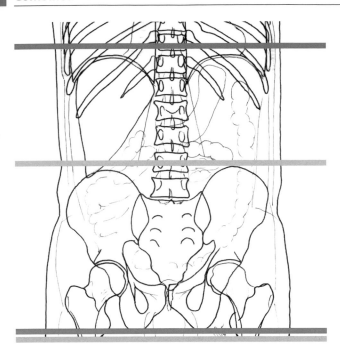

—— Slice boundaries for an abdominal examination
—— Slice boundaries for pelvic CT

Patient Preparation

– Fasting for 3 h (due to contrast administration)

Abdomen–pelvis:

– Approximately 60–90 min before the examination, fractionated oral administration of 1000 mL of CT-suitable contrast until just before the start of the examination (approx. 5 min before)
– Examination should be conducted with the bladder full (no bladder emptying before the examination, or catheter should be clamped)
– A vaginal tampon may be inserted if appropriate
– Rectal instillation of suitable contrast if appropriate
– Laboratory values (creatinine, baseline thyroid-stimulating hormone), allergy history, inquiry regarding renal and thyroid function, medication history

Materials

- 1000 mL CT-suitable contrast
- Rectal instillation of suitable contrast is possible (as a single enema = 200 mL or approx. 200–500 mL in a disposable colon bag with inflow tube)
- Hyoscine butylbromide (Buscopan) or glucagon can be injected to reduce intestinal peristalsis, with a 2-mL syringe and an 18-gauge needle (if an indwelling or butterfly catheter has not been placed)

Intravenous contrast if needed:

- 1 indwelling or butterfly catheter (16- or 18-gauge)
- 100 mL contrast (fill an injection syringe) or two 50 mL syringes filled with contrast (approximately 300 mg iodine/mL)
- Pressure dressing, swabs, skin disinfectant, adhesive bandages

▲ **Positioning**

- Supine, with the lower legs cushioned
- Arms folded behind the head

Parameters

- Scan range start: 1, dome of the diaphragm; 2, iliac crest
- Scan range end: 1, lower edge of the ischium; 2, lower edge of the ischium
- Breathing: breath held in inspiration
- Digital scout view: AP (512 mm)
- Scanning unit tilt: 0
- Scan direction: craniocaudal
- Documentation, soft-tissue window:
  WL: 40–60 HU
  WW: 200–500 HU

Type/ orientation		Collima- tion (pa- rameters)	Speed	Pitch factor	Slice thickness	Scanning param- eters (kV)
For all						
1	Topo AP (lat)	1–3 mm				100–130
1	Topo AP (cor) long (512 mm)	1–3 mm				100–130
Contrast medium application		Amount: 100–120 mL		Flow: 1.5–3 mL/s		Delay: 50–30 s
Postcontrast:						
1-line						
2	Abdominal spiral, axial	(7) 8 mm	(7.5) 12.8	1.5–1.6	(7) 8 mm	110–130
Immediately after:						
3	Pelvic spiral, axial	(7) 8 mm	(7.5) 12.8	1.5–1.6	(7) 8 mm	110–130
2-line						
2	Abdominal spiral, axial	[2×] 5 mm	20	2	5–8 mm	110–130
3	Pelvic spiral, axial	[2×] 4 mm	16	2	3.5–5 mm	110–130
6-line						
2	Abdominal spiral, axial	[6×] 2 mm	10	0.85	5–6 mm	120–130
3	Pelvic spiral, axial	[6×] 1 mm	9	1.5	1.25–3 mm	120–130
16-line						
2	Abdominal spiral, axial	[16×] 1.5–2 mm	24–36	1.0–1.5	4–5 mm	120–130
3	Pelvic spiral, axial	[16×] 1.5–2 mm	24–36	1.0–1.5	1.25–3 mm	120–130
64-line						
2	Abdominal spiral, axial	[64×] 0.6 mm	26.9	1.4	5 mm	120
3	Pelvic spiral, axial	[64×] 0.6 mm	26.9	1.4	5 mm	120

Non-contrast	For specific investigations (e. g., calculus), noncontrast imaging can be carried out before contrast administration either as a pelvic or abdominal study

! Tips & Tricks

- When specific issues are being investigated (e.g., tumors, diverticulitis, ureteral processes), pelvic spirals (e.g., with late imaging) can be carried out with the patient in the prone position (this provides better assessment of tumor infiltration and the spread of inflammation)
- A dilute barium solution (1–2%), water-soluble contrast containing iodine (2–4%), or simply water can be used as oral contrast media. For investigations of the stomach and bowel, focal lesions in the kidney, and CT angiography, water is actually better
- Negative contrast of the intestines is also possible (with instillation of cooking oil—e.g., for investigating the colon)
- Late imaging can be carried out if there is poor bowel contrast or after intravenous contrast injection—e.g., if there is a questionable renal or bladder process, and to demonstrate the ureters
- In spiral CT involving longer examination times, patients should be asked to hyperventilate before the spiral (caution is needed here in older patients), or should be allowed to breathe out slowly
- If there is known cardiac insufficiency, the delay can be extended
- If there are "poor" veins, reduce the flow (rule of thumb:
  flow –0.5 mL = delay + 10 s)
- The reconstruction increment for coronal and sagittal reconstructions should be approximately 70% of the reconstructed slice thickness

Caution:

- In patients with pheochromocytoma, intravenous contrast administration can trigger a hypertensive crisis
- If a possible intestinal stenosis is being investigated, only water or a water-soluble contrast medium should be used

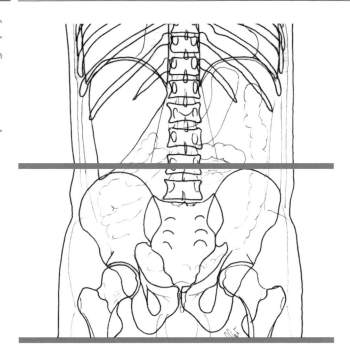

—— Slice boundaries for pelvic CT

Patient Preparation

– Fasting for 3 h (due to contrast administration)
– Laboratory values (creatinine, baseline thyroid-stimulating hormone), allergy history, inquiry regarding renal and thyroid function, medication history
– Examination should be conducted with the bladder full (no bladder emptying before the examination, or catheter should be clamped)
– Approximately 60–90 min before the examination, fractionated oral administration of 1000 mL of CT-suitable contrast
– A vaginal tampon may be inserted for women
– Rectal instillation of suitable warmed contrast if appropriate (approx. 500 mL in a disposable colon bag with inflow tube or 150 mL as a single enema)

Materials

- 1000 mL CT-suitable contrast
- Rectal instillation of suitable contrast is possible (as a single enema =200 mL or approx. 200–500 mL in a disposable colon bag with inflow tube)
- Hyoscine butylbromide (Buscopan) or glucagon can be injected to reduce intestinal peristalsis, with a 2-mL syringe and an 18-gauge needle (if an indwelling or butterfly catheter has not been placed)

Intravenous contrast if needed:

- 1 indwelling or butterfly catheter (16- or 18-gauge)
- 100 mL contrast (fill an injection syringe) or two 50-mL syringes filled with contrast (approximately 300 mg iodine/mL)
- Pressure dressing, swabs, skin disinfectant, adhesive bandages

▲ Positioning

- Supine, with the lower legs cushioned
- Arms folded behind the head

Parameters

- Scan range start: iliac crest
- Scan range end: lower edge of the ischium
- Breathing: breath-holding not usually needed (or breath held in expiration)
- Digital scout view: AP (512 mm)
- Scanning unit tilt: 0
- Scan direction: craniocaudal
- Documentation, soft-tissue window:
  WL: 40–60 HU
  WW: 200–500 HU

Type/ orientation		Collimation (parameters)	Speed	Pitch factor	Slice thickness	Scanning parameters (kV)
For all						
1	Topo AP (cor) long (512 mm)	1–3 mm				100–130
Contrast medium application		Amount: 100–120 mL		Flow: 1.5–3 mL/s		Delay: 50–30 s
Postcontrast:						
1-line						
2	Pelvic spiral, axial	(7) 8 mm	(7.5) 12.8	1.5–1.6	(7) 8 mm	130
2-line						
2	Pelvic spiral, axial	[2×] 5 mm	15	1.5	5–8 mm	130
6-line						
2	Pelvic spiral, axial	[6×] 2 mm	18	1.5	5 mm	130
16-line						
2	Pelvic spiral, axial	[16×] 1.5–2 mm	24–36	1.0–1.5	4–5 mm	130
64-line						
2	Pelvic spiral, axial	[24×] 1.2 mm	25.9	0.9	4–5 mm	120
Non-contrast	For specific investigations (e. g., calcification, calculus), before contrast administration, otherwise as for pelvic spirals					
Late imaging	For specific investigations (e. g., diverticulitis, tumors, ureter), wait 5–15 min after contrast administration; otherwise as for pelvic spirals (n. b.: full bladder; can be carried out with the patient in prone position)					

❗ Tips & Tricks

- When specific issues are being investigated (e.g., tumors, diverticulitis, ureteral processes), late imaging can be carried out with the patient in the prone position (this provides better assessment of tumor infiltration and the spread of inflammation)
- A dilute barium solution (1–2%), water-soluble contrast containing iodine (2–4%), or simply water can be used as oral contrast media. For investigations of the stomach and bowel, focal lesions in the kidney, and CT angiography, water is actually better
- Negative contrast of the intestines is also possible (with instillation of cooking oil—e.g., for investigating the colon)
- Late imaging can be carried out if there is poor bowel contrast or after intravenous contrast injection—e.g., if there is a questionable renal or bladder process
- If there is known cardiac insufficiency, the delay can be extended
- If there are "poor" veins, reduce the flow (rule of thumb:
  flow –0.5 mL = delay + 10 s)
- The reconstruction increment for coronal and sagittal reconstructions should be approximately 70% of the reconstructed slice thickness

Caution:
- In patients with pheochromocytoma, intravenous contrast administration can trigger a hypertensive crisis
- If a possible intestinal stenosis is being investigated, only water or a water-soluble contrast medium should be used

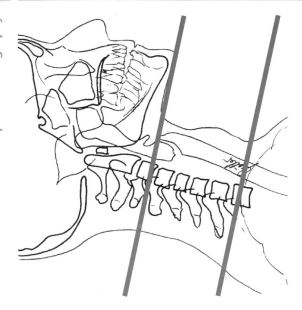

—— Slice boundaries for cervical CT

▨ Patient Preparation

– Radiography of the cervical spine at two levels may be needed
– Patient should be asked about previous spinal injuries (before positioning)

▲ Positioning

– Supine, with the neck slightly stretched
– Arms along the sides of the body, shoulders should be pulled down if appropriate (e.g., with aids: holding a rope that passes round the feet will pull the wrists downward)
– Head immobilized

Parameters

- Scan range start: according to clinical details (e.g., C4–T1 prolapse)
- Scan range end: according to clinical details
- Breathing: breath held in inspiration, no swallowing
- Digital scout view: lateral (256 mm)
- Scanning unit tilt: 0 or parallel to the intervertebral disk, then continuous
- Scan direction: craniocaudal
- Documentation:
  Soft-tissue window:
  WL: 30–40 HU
  WW: 200–300 HU
  Bone window if appropriate:
  WL: 200–500 HU
  WW: 1000–1800 HU
  For fracture examinations: multiplanar reconstruction
- Reconstruction: soft-tissue filter, possibly bone filter (core)

Type/ orientation	Collimation (parameters)	Speed	Pitch factor	Reconstruction increment	Scanning parameters (kV)
For all					
1	Lateral scout (256 mm)	2–4 mm			120
1-line					
2	Cervical spiral, axial	1.5–2 mm	1.5–2	1	1.5–2 mm	130–140
2-line					
2	Cervical spiral, axial	[2 ×] 1.5 mm	3	1	3 (1.5) mm	130
6-line					
2	Cervical spiral, axial	[6 ×] 1 mm	4.8–9	0.8 (1.5)	2 (0.8) mm	130
16-line					
2	Cervical spiral, axial	[16 ×] 0.75 mm	6–9	0.5–0.75	2–3 mm	130
64-line					
2	Cervical spiral, axial	[64 ×] 0.6 mm	17.3	0.9	2 (0.75) mm	130

Variation

Contrast CT of the cervical spine (e.g., for investigating tumor)
Preparation
– Fasting for 3 hours only with contrast administration
– Creatinine, thyroid values (baseline thyroid-stimulating hormone); patient must be provided with information about contrast administration
Materials
– 1 indwelling or butterfly catheter (16- or 18-gauge)
– Pressure dressing, swabs, skin disinfectant, adhesive bandages
– 1 indwelling or butterfly catheter (16- or 18-gauge)
– 100 mL contrast (approximately 300 mg iodine/mL), fill an injection syringe (or two 50-mL syringes filled with contrast; manual bolus injection approx. 30 s before the start of scanning)
– Injection parameters: 2–3 mL/s; delay 40–70 s; then cervical spirals (see above)

Tips & Tricks

- The shoulder girdle should be pulled downward as much as possible (the patient can hold the ends of a rope with both hands—e.g., using loops at the top—and the middle of the rope can be passed under the soles of the feet so that the shoulders are pulled downward when the legs are stretched out)
- With multiplanar devices, three reconstruction processes are documented: axial soft-tissue filter, sagittal soft-tissue filter, and sagittal bone filter (core), each with the appropriate window (see above)
- To improve the image quality, the collimation, reconstruction increment, and slice thickness can be reduced

Computed Tomography

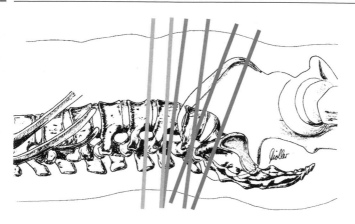

≡ Slice boundaries for lumbar CT parallel to the intervertebral disk

Patient Preparation

- Radiography of the lumbar spine at two levels may be needed
- Fasting for 3 h only needed for contrast administration—e. g., after intervertebral disk surgery, and in these cases laboratory tests are also needed (creatinine, baseline thyroid-stimulating hormone), allergy history, inquiry regarding renal and thyroid function
- Patient should be asked about previous spinal injuries (before positioning)

Materials

- 1 indwelling or butterfly catheter (16- or 18-gauge)
- Injection syringe filled with 100 mL contrast (approximately 300 mg iodine/mL)
- Pressure dressing, swabs, skin disinfectant, adhesive bandages

Positioning

- Supine
- Arms folded behind the head or crossed on the chest
- Lumbar lordosis should be compensated during lumbar CT (using a knee cushion or a wedge cushion under the pelvis)

Parameters

Sequence mode in spiral CT (e.g., when investigating prolapse):
- Scan range start: according to clinical details (e.g., L3)
- Scan range end: according to clinical details (e.g., S1)

- Breathing: breath held, or shallow breathing
- Digital scout view: lateral (512 mm; 256 mm is often sufficient for lumbar imaging)
- Scanning unit tilt: Parallel to each intervertebral disk or top of each vertebra (e.g., L3/L4 = 0°, L4/L5 = +5°, L5/S1 = +15°)
- Scan direction: craniocaudal
- Documentation:
  Soft-tissue window (for images reconstructed in soft-tissue filter [core]):
  WL: 30–40 HU
  WW: 200–300 HU
  Bone window if appropriate (for images reconstructed in bone window [core]):
  WL: 200–500 HU
  WW: 1000–1800 HU

Type/ orientation		Collimation (parameters)	Speed	Slice thickness	Scanning parameters (kV)
For all					
1	Lateral scout (512 mm)	1–3 mm			120–140
1-line					
2	Lumbar sequence, axial*	3 mm	3	3 mm	130–140
2-line					
2	Lumbar sequence, axial*	[2 ×] 1.5 mm	3	3 mm	130
6-line					
2	Lumbar sequence, axial*	[6 ×] 1 mm	6	2 mm	130
16-line					
2	Lumbar sequence, axial*	[12–16 ×] 0.6–0.75 mm	7.2–9	1.5 mm	120–130
64-line					
2	Lumbar sequence, axial	[24 ×] 1.2 mm	28.5	1.5–2.4 mm	120–130

* Each axial lumbar sequence is angled over the corresponding segment.

Variations

Myelo-CT

Preparation:
- Patient information, written informed consent (for myelo-CT)

Materials:
- Spinal needle (atraumatic)
- 10-mL syringe with 10 mL contrast suitable for intrathecal administration
- Drape with opening, gloves, swabs
- Skin disinfection spray
- Contrast (for additional injections)
- Sterile tube (for cerebrospinal fluid examination)
- Foam wedge cushion

Positioning:
- Patient in lateral decubitus, knees drawn up tight
- Neck bent (chin on the chest)

Puncture:
- Puncture of the vertebral canal, usually at the L3/L4 level (or L4/L5)
- Aspiration of cerebrospinal fluid for cytological examination
- Injection of the contrast (injection speed 10 mL/60 s)
- At the end of the injection, the needle is removed and the recumbent patient should rotate once round his or her own axis

Documentation:
- Window level: 40–60 HU (or higher at stronger contrast concentrations)
- Window width: 400–500 HU (up to 2000 HU at stronger contrast concentrations)

Follow-up:
- 24 h bed rest
- Head should be raised for approx. 8 h (body position otherwise indifferent)
- Increased fluid intake (approx. 2–3 L)
- In case of headache (due to low cerebrospinal fluid pressure, usually on the day after the procedure): patient should lie flat, no analgesia initially

Contrast CT of the lumbar spine (e.g., for investigating tumor, recurrent prolapse, or postoperative scar)

Materials:
- 1 indwelling or butterfly catheter (16- or 18-gauge)
- Pressure dressing, swabs, skin disinfectant, adhesive bandages

– 100 mL contrast (approximately 300 mg iodine/mL), fill an injection syringe (or in two 50-mL syringes; bolus injection approx. 30 s before the start of scanning)
– Injection parameters: 2.5 mL/s; delay 50–70 s

❗ Tips & Tricks

– Sagittal reconstruction over the pathological finding (reconstruction in the soft-tissue filter [core], or bone filter [core], corresponding to what is documented in the soft-tissue and bone windows)
– A scout view (topogram) should be photographed alongside after each change of level, so that the slice level can be better visualized
– The corresponding vertebral levels should each be labeled (L4, L5, or in the intervertebral space L4/L5)
– Document the scout view with all scans taken at the end
– In lumbar CT after conventional myelography, a waiting period of 4–6 h should be observed after the injection, since otherwise the contrast is too high in the vertebral canal (leading to artifacts). The patient can be rolled once onto the stomach and back to distribute the contrast before the examination
– A reference scan should be carried out for each segment in order to adjust the size. The abdominal aorta is visible in the mid-lumbar spine, and the iliosacral joins should be visible at the level of L5/S1
– To improve the image quality, the collimation, reconstruction increment, and slice thickness can be reduced

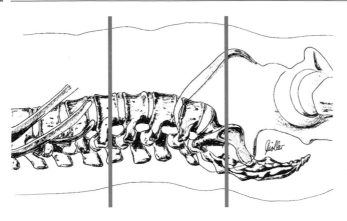

—— Slice boundaries for lumbar CT spiral

■ Patient Preparation
- Radiography of the lumbar spine (or thoracic spine) at two levels may be needed
- Patient should be asked about previous spinal injuries

▲ Positioning
- Supine
- Arms folded behind the head or crossed on the chest
- Lumbar lordosis should be compensated during lumbar CT (using a knee cushion or a wedge cushion under the pelvis)

Parameters
Spiral mode (for demonstrating the vertebrae, e.g., when investigating fractures and/or disk prolapse):
- Scan range start: according to clinical details
- Scan range end: according to clinical details
- Breathing: breath held, or shallow breathing
- Digital scout view: lateral (512 mm; 256 mm is often sufficient for lumbar imaging)
- Scanning unit tilt: 0 (in older devices, leave the gantry tilt at 0° to allow reconstruction), or parallel to the top of the vertebra of interest, then continuous
- Scan direction: craniocaudal

- Documentation:
  Bone window:
  WL: 200–500 HU
  WW: 1000–1800 HU
- Soft-tissue window if appropriate:
  WL: 30–40 HU
  WW: 200–300 HU
- Reconstruction: in the soft-tissue and bone filters (core), in accordance with the documentation in the soft-tissue and bone windows

Type/ orientation		Collimation (param- eters)	Speed	Pitch factor	Slice thickness	Scanning param- eters (kV)
For all						
1	Lateral scout (512 or 256 mm)	1–3 mm				120–140
1-line						
2	Lumbar se- quence, axial	3 mm	3	1	3 mm	130–140
2-line						
2	Lumbar se- quence, axial	[2×] 2.5 mm	5	1	3 mm	130
6-line						
2	Lumbar se- quence, axial	[6×] 2 mm	6–9	0.5–0.75	3 (1.5) mm	130
16-line						
2	Lumbar se- quence, axial	[16×] 0.6– 0.75 mm	6–9	0.5–0.75	1.5–3 mm	120–130
64-line						
2	Lumbar se- quence, axial	[64×] 0.6 mm	17.3	0.9	1.5–3 mm	120–130

Variations

Myelo-CT

Depending on issue being investigated, myelo-CT can be used (for technique, see CT of the Lumbar Spine, above)

Contrast CT of the lumbar spine (e. g., for investigating tumor)

Preparation:
– Fasting for 3 h only needed for contrast administration

Materials:
– 1 indwelling or butterfly catheter (16- or 18-gauge)
– Pressure dressing, swabs, skin disinfectant, adhesive bandages
– 100 mL contrast (approximately 300 mg iodine/mL), fill an injection syringe (or in two 50-mL syringes; manual bolus injection approx. 30 s before the start of scanning)
– Injection parameters: 2–3 mL/s; delay 40–70 s

! Tips & Tricks

– Sagittal and coronal reconstruction over the pathological finding (documentation in the soft-tissue and bone windows)
– Tilted reconstructions parallel to the intervertebral disk or top of vertebra
– The corresponding vertebral levels should each be labeled (L4, L5, or in the intervertebral space L4/L5)
– Document the scout view with all scans taken at the end
– In lumbar CT after conventional myelography, a waiting period of 4–6 h should be observed after the injection, since otherwise the contrast is too high in the vertebral canal (leading to artifacts). The patient can be rolled once onto the stomach and back to distribute the contrast before the examination
– To improve the image quality, the collimation, reconstruction increment, and slice thickness can be reduced

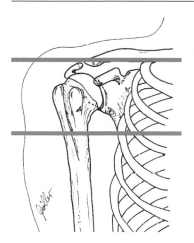 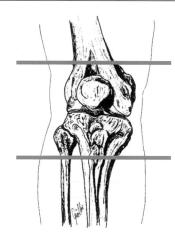

—— Slice boundaries for shoulder joint CT   —— Slice boundaries for knee joint CT

Patient Preparation

– Radiographic examination of the extremity or joint

Positioning

– Shoulder joint: supine, healthy arm above the head, arm on the side being examined alongside the body and positioned centrally. The healthy side should also have cushions placed underneath. (Alternative: both arms alongside the body, allowing bilateral comparison)
– Upper extremity (elbow, hand): prone, hand stretched out forward (preferably in supination for elbow joint examination), bilateral examination possible (e.g., of the hands) alongside for comparison
– Lower extremity: supine, healthy leg angled if possible, feet first

Parameters

Spiral CT

– Scan range start: according to clinical details (e.g., at the upper edge of the acromioclavicular joint or upper edge of the patella)
– Scan range end: according to clinical details (e.g., tip of the scapula or lower edge of the tibial condyle)
– Breathing: breath held for shoulder, otherwise quiet normal breathing possible
– Digital scout view: AP or lateral (256 mm)

- Scanning unit tilt: 0
- Scan direction: craniocaudal
- Reconstructions: coronal and sagittal, in the soft-tissue and bone filters (core)
- Documentation:
  Soft-tissue window:
  WL: 30–50 HU
  WW: 200–400 HU
  Bone window:
  WL: 200–500 HU
  WW: 1400–1800 HU

Type/ orientation		Collimation (parameters)	Speed	Pitch factor	Slice thickness	Scanning parameters (kV)
For all						
1	Scout view AP or lateral (256 mm)	1–3 mm				100–130
1-line						
2	Extremity, axial	1.5–2 mm	3–5	1.5–2	2 mm	120–130
2-line						
2	Extremity, axial	[2×] 1 mm	2	1	3 (1) mm	120–130
6-line						
2	Extremity, axial	[6×] 1 mm	9	1.5	5 (0.8) mm	120–130
16-line						
2	Extremity, axial	[16×] 0.6–0.75 mm	6–14.4	0.5–1.5	1.5 mm	120–130
64-line						
2	Extremity, axial	[64×] 0.6 mm	3.2	0.9	3 (0.6) mm	120

Variations

Contrast CT of the extremity (e. g., for investigating tumor)

Materials:
- 1 indwelling or butterfly catheter (16- or 18-gauge)
- Pressure dressing, swabs, skin disinfectant, adhesive bandages
- 100 mL contrast (approximately 300 mg iodine/mL), fill an injection syringe (or in two 50-mL syringes; bolus injection, delay approx. 20–30 s)
- Injection parameters: 2–3 mL/s; delay 40–70 s

CT arthrography (e. g., shoulder joint)

Materials:
- Sterile table
- 1 10-mL syringe with 18-gauge needle (for anesthesia)
- 1 5-mL syringe (with contrast, 3–5 mL, approx. 300 mg iodine/mL)
- 1 spinal needle, 22-gauge (black)
- 1 flexible plastic connection tube (approx. 20 cm long)
- Sterile drape with opening, sterile swabs, sterile gloves, skin disinfectant, local anesthetic, adhesive bandages

Positioning:
- Flat supine position, arms slightly abducted and externally rotated, skin disinfection, sterile draping

Puncture:
- Superficial skin anesthesia

Procedure:
- With CT guidance, marking of the injection site at approximately the center of the articular cavity
- During constant slow injection of local anesthetic, vertical puncture of the articular cavity from the ventral position
- Intra-articular injection of 3–5 mL contrast
- Withdrawal of the catheter
- Active and passive movement exercises until even distribution is achieved

! Tips & Tricks
- Sagittal reconstruction over the pathological finding (documentation in the bone and soft-tissue windows)
- When positioning the extremities, attention should be given to good, stable cushioning
- Sagittal and coronal reconstructions over the pathological finding

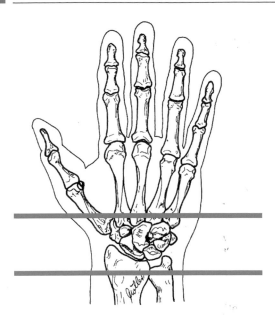

——— Slice boundaries for wrist CT

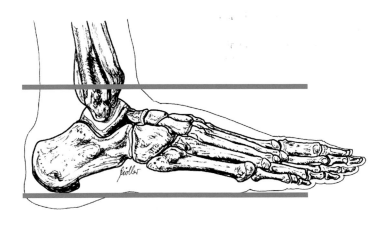

——— Slice boundaries for foot CT

■ **Patient Preparation**

– Radiographic examination of the extremity or joint

▲ **Positioning**

– Upper extremity (e.g., hand): prone, hand stretched out forward, bilateral examination alongside for comparison possible
– Lower extremity: supine, healthy leg angled if possible, feet first (n.b.: for comparative studies, ensure symmetrical positioning and place the two joints as close together as possible—this allows the field of view to be kept as small as possible)

Parameters

Spiral CT

– Scan range start: according to clinical details (e.g., distal radius)
– Scan range end: according to clinical details (e.g., distal metacarpal ends)
– Breathing: quiet normal breathing
– Digital scout view: AP or lateral (256 mm)
– Scanning unit tilt: 0
– Scan direction: craniocaudal
– Reconstructions: coronal and sagittal in the bone filter (core); for specific issues (e.g. soft-tissue tumor), soft-tissue filter as well (core)
– Documentation:
  Soft-tissue window:
  WL: 30–50 HU
  WW: 200–400 HU
  Bone window:
  WL: 200–500 HU
  WW: 1400–1800 HU

Type/ orientation		Collima- tion (pa- rameters)	Speed	Pitch factor	Slice thickness	Scanning param- eters (kV)
For all						
1	Scout view AP or lateral (256 mm)	1–3 mm				100–130
1-line						
2	Extremity, axial	1.5–3 mm	3–5	1.5–2	2 mm	120–130
2-line						
2	Extremity, axial	[2×] 1 mm	2	1	2 (0.8) mm	120–130
6-line						
2	Extremity, axial	[6×] 0.5– 0.75 mm	2.4–4.5	1–0.8	2 (0.6) mm	120–130
16-line						
2	Extremity, axial	[2–4×] 0.6 mm	0.8–1.8	0.65– 0.75	2 (0.5) mm	120–130
64-line						
2	Extremity, axial	[12×] 0.6 (0.3) mm	3.2	0.9	2 (0.2–0.4) mm	120–130

! Tips & Tricks

- Sagittal reconstruction over the pathological finding (reconstruction depending on the issue being investigated, with bone and soft-tissue filters (core—e.g., bone/sharp), documentation in the bone and soft-tissue windows)
- When positioning the extremities, attention should be given to good, stable cushioning
- Sagittal and coronal reconstructions over the pathological finding
- To improve the image quality, the collimation, reconstruction increment, and slice thickness can be reduced
- Depending on the issue being investigated, particularly in 1-line scans, the calcaneus or metatarsals can be tilted for better secondary reconstruction

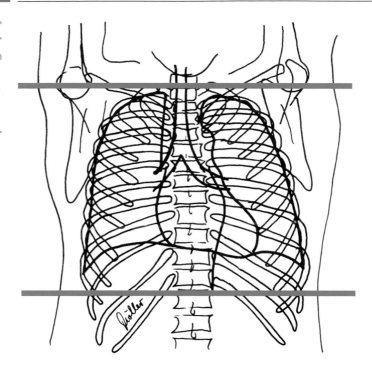

—— Slice boundaries for CT angiography of the thoracic aorta

Patient Preparation

– Fasting for 3 h if possible (due to contrast administration)
– Laboratory values (creatinine, baseline thyroid-stimulating hormone), allergy history, inquiry regarding renal and thyroid function, medication history

Materials

– 1 indwelling catheter (16-gauge)
– 100–120 mL contrast (fill an injection syringe; ca. 300–370 mg iodine/mL)
– Pressure dressing, swabs, skin disinfectant, adhesive bandages

▲ **Positioning**

– Symmetrical supine position, lower legs cushioned
– Gonads shielded
– Arms stretched up over the head (or folded behind the head)

Parameters

– Scan range start: lowest costal arch
– Scan range end: apex of the chest
– Breathing: breath held in inspiration
– Digital scout view: AP (512 mm)
– Scan direction: caudocranial (also craniocaudal from 16-line up)
– Documentation: MPR, MIP, VTR, vessel analysis

Type/ orientation	Collimation (parameters)	Speed	Pitch factor	Slice thickness	Scanning parameters (kV)
For all					
1	Scout view AP (512 mm)	1–3 mm				100–130
Contrast medium application	Amount: 100–120 mL	Flow: 3–4 mL/s			Bolus tracking (trigger level at 120 HU if ROI in aortic arch)
2-line					
2	Abdominal spiral, axial	[2×] 2.5 mm	10	2	5 mm	110–120
6-line					
2	Abdominal spiral, axial	[6×] 1 mm	9	1.5	5 mm	110–120
16-line					
2	Abdominal spiral, axial	[16×] 0.75–1 mm	12–18	1.0–1.5	3–5 mm	110–120
64-line					
2	Abdominal spiral, axial	[64×] 0.6 mm	23	1.0–1.5	5 (0.75) mm	110–120

ROI, region of interest.

❗ Tips & Tricks

– In spiral CT involving longer examination times, patients should be asked to hyperventilate before the spiral (caution is needed here in older patients)
– Breathing commands should be explained to the patient beforehand and practiced
– Feet first in intensive-care patients makes positioning easier
– To improve reconstruction, thin slices can be selected for reconstruction and a reconstruction increment smaller than the slice thickness can be selected (overlapping)

Caution:

– In patients with pheochromocytoma, intravenous contrast administration can trigger a hypertensive crisis

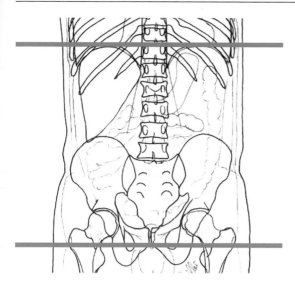

—— Slice boundaries for CT angiography of the abdominal aorta

▧ Patient Preparation

- Fasting for 3 h (due to contrast administration)
- Laboratory values (creatinine, baseline thyroid-stimulating hormone), allergy history, inquiry regarding renal and thyroid function, medication history
- No oral contrast; if contrast is needed, then fractionated administration of 1000 mL orally approx. 60–90 min before the examination

Materials

- 1 indwelling or butterfly catheter (16-gauge)
- 100–120 mL contrast (fill an injection syringe; ca. 300–370 mg iodine/mL)
- Pressure dressing, swabs, skin disinfectant, adhesive bandages

▲ Positioning

- Supine, lower legs cushioned
- Arms folded behind the head

Parameters

– Scan range start: dome of the diaphragm
– Scan range end: approx. upper edge of ischium
– Breathing: breath held in inspiration
– Digital scout view: AP (512 mm)
– Scanning unit tilt: 0
– Scan direction: craniocaudal
– Documentation: MIP, 3D, VTR, vessel analysis

Type/ orientation		Collimation (parameters)	Speed	Pitch factor	Slice thickness	Scanning pa-rameters (kV)
For all						
1	Scout view AP (512 mm)	1–3 mm				100–130
Contrast medium application		Amount: 100–120 mL		Flow: 3–4 mL/s		Bolus tracking (trigger level at 120 HU if ROI in aortic arch) or delay 25–30 s
2-line						
2	Abdominal spiral, axial	[2×] 1.5 mm	6	2	5 mm	110–120
6-line						
2	Abdominal spiral, axial	[6×] 1 mm	9	1.5	5 mm	110–120
16-line						
2	Abdominal spiral, axial	[16×] 0.625–1 mm	9–18	1.0–1.5	3–5 mm	110–120
64-line						
2	Abdominal spiral, axial	[16×] 0.6 mm	23	1.0–1.5	(0.75) 5 mm	110–120

Tips & Tricks

– In spiral CT involving longer examination times, patients should be asked to hyperventilate before the spiral (caution is needed here in older patients)
– Breathing commands should be explained to the patient beforehand and practiced
– Feet first in intensive-care patients makes positioning easier
– To improve reconstruction, thin slices can be selected for reconstruction and a reconstruction increment smaller than the slice thickness can be selected (overlapping)

Caution:

– In patients with pheochromocytoma, intravenous contrast administration can trigger a hypertensive crisis

Magnetic Resonance Imaging

Cranial MRI

Patient Preparation

- Patient should visit the rest room before the examination
- Patient should be given information about the procedure and should be offered ear protection (e.g. ear plugs)
- Any metal items should be removed (dentures, hearing aids, hairpins, piercing, earrings, etc.)
- An indwelling catheter may be placed (e.g., if tumor or multiple sclerosis need to be investigated)

▲ Positioning

- Supine
- Head should be immobilized in the head coil
- Cushions placed under the legs

Sequences

- Scout: sagittal and transverse (best with three levels)
1. *Transverse sequence:* mark on the mid-sagittal, line through anterior and posterior end of the bar (parallel to a line through the anterior and posterior commissure); do as many slices as need to fully image the brain from the vertex to the cerebellum
- T2 (example: tse TR: 3500–4500, TE 100–120)
- Slice thickness: 5–6 mm
- Interslice interval: 1.2
- Matrix: 512

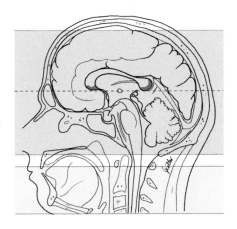

Transverse neurocranium, 1st and 2nd sequences

– Saturation: parallel to the slices, block underneath the lowest slice (50–80 mm)
2. *Transverse sequence:* orientation, slice thickness and slice position as in sequence 1
– T1 (example: SE, TR: 450–600, TE: 12–25 or FFE: TR: as short as possible, TE: 12, pulse angle 30°)
– Slice thickness: 6 mm
– Interslice interval: 1.2
– Saturation: parallel to slices, block underneath the lowest slice (50–80 mm)
 Or: 1st + 2nd sequence as double echo (T2/protons; example: TR 3000–4500, TE 100/15)
3. *Coronal sequence* (perpendicular to 1)
– FLAIR (example: 1.5 Tesla: TR 9000, TE 120, TI 2300; 1.0 or 0.5 T: TR 5000, TE 100, TI 1900)
– Slice thickness: 6 mm
– Interslice interval: 1.2
– Saturation: perpendicular to the slices (transverse over the neck)

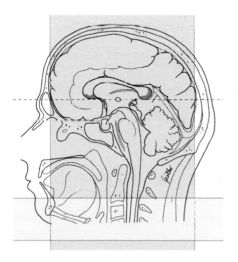

Coronal neurocranium,
3 rd sequence

4. *Sagittal sequence:*
– T2 (example: tse TR 3500–4500, TE 100–120 or FFE: TR 900, TE 27, pulse angle 15°
– Slice thickness: 5–6 mm
– Interslice interval: 1.2
– Saturation: perpendicular to the slices (transverse over the neck)

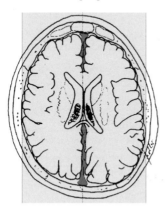

Sagittal neurocranium,
4th sequence

! **Tips & Tricks**
– Symmetrical positioning: note the root of the nose
– Place cushions under the knees
– In patients with more rounded backs, place cushions under the pelvis; in those with cervical symptoms, the head can be raised and cushioned

Excluding Hemorrhage

Sequences 1–4: as above
5. *Coronal sequence* (= perpendicular to 1) or *transverse* (orientation as for sequence 1)
– T2 gradient echo (example: 1.5 T: FLASH: TR 800, TE 15/35, pulse angle 20°; 0.5 T: FFE: TR 900, TE 27, pulse angle 15°)
– Slice thickness: 5–6 mm
– Interslice interval: 1.3
– Saturation: perpendicular to the slices (transverse over the neck)

Postoperative Neurocranium (after Tumor Surgery)

■ **Patient Preparation**

– An indwelling catheter with an extension tube should be placed

1. *Transverse sequence* T2 (as above, basic sequence 1)
2. *Transverse sequence* T1 (as above, basic sequence 2)
3. *Transverse sequence* T1: exactly as in sequence 2, but after contrast administration (e. g., Gd-DTPA)
4. *Coronal sequence* T1, otherwise as in sequence 2, but after contrast administration
5. *Sagittal sequence* T1, otherwise as in sequence 2, but after contrast administration

Inner Ear (e. g., Vestibular Schwannoma)

■ **Patient Preparation**

– An indwelling catheter with an extension tube should be placed
1. *Coronal sequence* FLAIR
– As above, basic sequence 3
2. *Transverse sequence*
– T2 (example: tse TR 3500–4500, TE 100–120)
– Slice thickness: 3 mm
– Interslice interval: 1.2 (or 1 mm)
– Saturation: parallel to slices, block underneath lowest slice (50–80 mm)

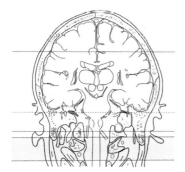

Transverse inner ear, sequence 2

3. *Transverse sequence* (mark on coronal slice)
- T1 (example: SE, TR 450–600, TE 12–25 or FFE: TR, as short as possible, TE 12, pulse angle 30°)
- Slice thickness: 0.8–1.5 mm
- Interslice interval: 1.0
- Saturation: parallel to slices, block underneath lowest slice and above the uppermost slice

Transverse inner ear, sequence 3

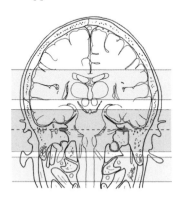

4. *Transverse sequence:* exactly as in sequence 3, but after contrast administration (e.g., Gd-DTPA)

Possible 5th *transverse sequence*
- 3D T2 high-resolution (example: CISS TR: 12.25, TE 5.9, pulse angle 90°, block thickness 30–35 mm, partitions 40–50, FOV 180–200)

Epilepsy (Temporal Lobe Adjustment)
- Scout: see above
- 2nd scout: sagittal over the temporal lobe

1. *Transverse sequence* T2 (see above, basic sequence 1)
2. *Coronal sequence* FLAIR (see above, basic sequence 3)
3. *Transverse sequence* (mark on temporal lobe scout: parallel to the course of the temporal lobe)
- T2 (example: tse TR 3500–4500, TE 100–120)
- Slice thickness: 3 mm
- Interslice interval: 1.0
- Saturation: parallel to the slices, block underneath the lowest slice

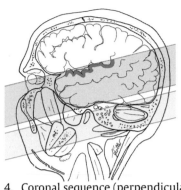

Epilepsy (temporal lobe), transverse, sequence 3

4. Coronal sequence (perpendicular to the slices in sequence 3, only over the temporal lobe and the temporal lobe apex)
   - Turbo inversion recovery (TIR) (example: 1.5 T, TR 7000, TE 60, TI 400; 0.5 T, TR 2850, TE 20, TI 400)
   - Slice thickness: 3 mm
   - Interslice interval: 1.5
   - Saturation: no

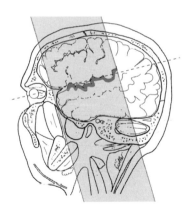

Epilepsy (temporal lobe), coronal, sequence 4

Orbit

▮ Patient Preparation
- An indwelling catheter with an extension tube should be placed
- Patient should close the eyes during the examination
-

1. *Transverse sequence* T2 (see above, basic sequence 1)
2. *Transverse sequence*
   - T1, fat-saturated (example: SE TR 500–600, TE 12–25; 0.5 T, FFE: TR as short as possible, TE 6–12, pulse angle 30°)
   - Slice thickness: 4–5 mm
   - Interslice interval: 1.2
   - Saturation: parallel to the slices, block underneath the lowest and above the uppermost slice

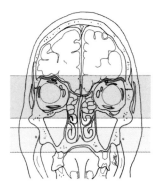

Transverse orbit, sequence 2

3. *Coronal sequence*
   - T2, fat-saturated (example: tse TR 3500–4500, TE 100–120)
   - Slice thickness: 4–5 mm
   - Interslice interval: 1.2
   - Saturation: no

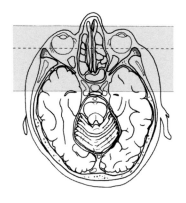

Coronal orbit, sequence 3

4. *Transverse sequence:* exactly as in sequence 3, but after contrast administration (e.g., Gd-DTPA)
5. *Parasagittal sequence* (along the optic nerve, mark on the transverse slice)
– T1 (example: SE, TR 450–600, TE 12–25)
– Slice thickness: 3 mm
– Interslice interval: 1.0
– Saturation: no

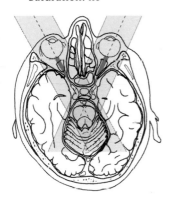

Parasagittal orbit, sequence 5

Sella

███ **Patient Preparation**

– An indwelling catheter with an extension tube should be placed
1. *Transverse sequence* T2 (see above, basic sequence 1)
2. *Coronal sequence* FLAIR (see above, basic sequence 3)
3. *Coronal sequence* (mark on mid-sagittal scout over the sella)
– T1 (example: SE, TR 500–600, TE 12 [1.5 T], 16 [1.0 T], 25 [0.5 T], pulse angle 90° for each)
or 3D FFE:
TR as short as possible, TE 6.9 (1.0 T), 12–13 (0.5 T), pulse angle 30° for each
– Slice thickness: 2 mm (1 mm overlapping possible)
– Interslice interval: 1.0
– Saturation: (a) perpendicular to the slices (transverse over the neck); (b) paracoronal behind the slices over the sinus
– FOV: small (e.g., 200 mm)

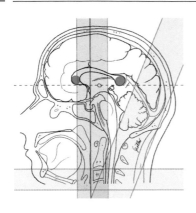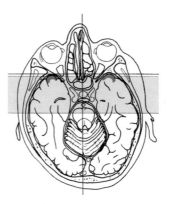

Coronal sella, sequence 3

4. *Coronal sequence:* exactly as in sequence 3, but after contrast administration (e. g., Gd-DTPA)
5. *Sagittal sequence* after contrast administration (e. g., Gd-DTPA) (mark on coronal scout above the sella)
– T1 (example: SE, TR 500, TE 12 [1.5 T], 16 [1.0 T], 25 [0.5 T], pulse angle 90° for each)
  or 3D FFE:
  TR as short as possible, TE 6.9 (1.0 T), 12–13 (0.5 T), pulse angle 30° for each
– Slice thickness: 2 mm (1 mm overlapping possible)
– Interslice interval: 1.0
– Saturation: coronal block over the posterior cranial fossa or sinus (since phase is posteroanterior)
– FOV: small (e. g., 200 mm)

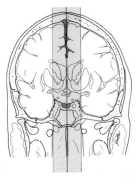
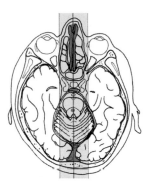

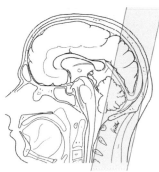

Sagittal sella postcontrast, sequence 5

Variant Examinations

- Sequence 4 can be made "dynamic" – i.e., keep TR short enough and the turbo factor high enough for the sequence to take 10–15 s. About 15 sequences in succession (example: TR 500, TE 13, turbo factor 7)
- Another noncontrast sagittal T1 sequence can be added between sequences 4 and 5 (as in sequence 5, but without contrast)

Magnetic Resonance Imaging

MRI of the Cervical Spine

■ **Patient Preparation**

– Patient should visit the rest room before the examination
– Patient should be given information about the procedure, with particular mention of how to avoid swallowing artifacts and motion artifacts (comfortable positioning, no pain)
– Ear protection (e.g. ear plugs) should be offered
– Any metal items should be removed (dentures, hearing aids, hairpins, piercing, etc.)
– An indwelling catheter may be placed (e.g., if tumor, multiple sclerosis, spondylodiskitis, or abscess need to be investigated)

▲ **Positioning**

– Supine on the cervical coil
– Cushions placed under the legs
– Arms alongside the body

Sequences

– Scout: sagittal and coronal (best with three levels)
1. *Sagittal sequence* (mark on coronal scout; as many slices as are necessary to fully image the spine)
– T2 (example: tse TR 3000–3500, TE 100–120)
– Slice thickness: 3–4 mm
– Interslice interval: 1.0
– Phase: FH with 100% oversampling due to wrap-around artifacts
– Saturation: coronal in front of (and possibly behind) the spine

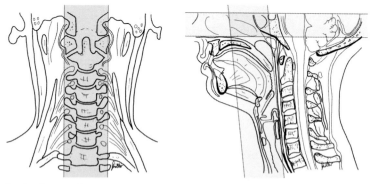

Sagittal cervical spine, sequences 1 and 2 (with additional transverse saturation)

2. *Sagittal sequence* (as sequence 1)
   - Protons (example: 1.5–0.5 T: tse, example: TR 1200–1700, TE 12–20) or T1 (example: tse TR 500, TE 15)
   - Phase: PA
   - Slice thickness and interval as in sequence 1
   - Saturation: (a) coronal in front of (and possibly behind) the spine; (b) transverse above; and possibly (c) transverse under the sagittal slices
   - Or sequence 1 + 2: sagittal double echo, otherwise as in sequence 1
3. *Transverse sequence* parallel to the corresponding vertebral surfaces (in a normal cervical spine, the same slice setting through from C 4 to T 1, for example, is usually sufficient)
   - Protons (example: tse TR 1700, TE 12) or T2 (example: gradient echo 1.5 T: TR 850, TE 26, pulse angle 30°; 0.5 T: TR 55, TE 27, pulse angle 6°)
   - Slice thickness: 3–4 mm
   - Interslice interval: 1.0
   - Phase-encoding direction: PA
   - Saturation: (a) coronal in front of the spine; (b) transverse (parallel to the slices) over the slice block; and (c) transverse (parallel to the slices) under the slice block
   - Or: motion artifact suppression; in this case only coronal saturation

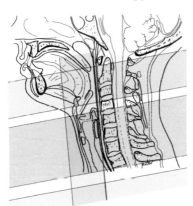

Transverse cervical spine, parallel to the corresponding vertebral surfaces, sequence 3

4. *Coronal sequence*
– T2 (example: tse with higher turbo factor—e. g., TR 3000–4000, TE 100–140)
– Slice thickness: 6 mm
– Interslice interval: 1.0
– Saturation: no

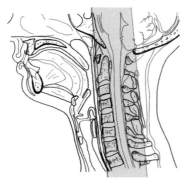

Coronal cervical spine, sequence 4

❗ Tips & Tricks

– In patients with more rounded backs, place cushions under the pelvis; in those with cervical symptoms, the head can be raised and cushioned
– The patient should swallow again and clear the throat before sequence 1
– If there is severe scoliosis, ensure that enough slices are used to include the lateral areas
– Adjustment aids (cervical spine): centering on the middle of the neck (or deeper in those with a short neck)

Suspected Tumor, Suspected Spondylodiskitis, Abscess

▮ Patient Preparation

– An indwelling catheter with an extension tube should be placed

1. *Sagittal sequence,* T2 (see above, basic sequence 1)
2. *Sagittal sequence* (as sequence 1)
– T1 (example: SE, TR 450–600, TE 12–25)
– Phase: AP
– Slice thickness, interval and saturation as in sequence 2
3. *Transverse sequence* (through the region of interest)
– T1 (example: tse TR 450–600, TE 10–25)
– Slice thickness: 4 mm

- Interslice interval: 1.0
- Three saturators: (a) perpendicular (coronal) to the slices, block saturates the area of the spine; (b) transverse (parallel to the slices) over and (c) under the slice block
4. *Transverse sequence* T1: as sequence 3, but after contrast administration
5. *Sagittal sequence* T1: as sequence 2, but after contrast administration (e.g., Gd-DTPA)

Suspected Disseminated Encephalomyelitis or Syringomyelia

■ **Patient Preparation**
- An indwelling catheter with an extension tube should be placed

1. *Sagittal sequence* T2 (see above, basic sequence 1)
2. *Transverse sequence* (through the region of interest)
- T2 (example: gradient echo: 1.5T: TR 850, TE 26, pulse angle 30°; 0.5T: TR 55, TE 27, pulse angle 6°; or T2 TSE TR 3000, TE 130, pulse angle 90°)
- Slice thickness, interval and saturation as in sequence 3
3. *Sagittal sequence* (as in basic sequence 1)
- T1 (tse, example: TR 500–600, TE 12–15, pulse angle 90° or 150°)
- Slice thickness, interval and saturation as in sequence 2 above
4. *Sagittal sequence:* as in basic sequence 1), but after contrast administration (e.g., Gd-DTPA)

Trauma, Suspected Fracture

■ **Patient Preparation**
- An indwelling catheter with an extension tube may be placed

1. *Sagittal sequence*
- Turbo inversion recovery (TIRM) or spectral presaturation with inversion recovery (SPIR) (example: TR 6500, TE 30–60, TI 140, pulse angle 180°) or fat-saturated T2 (example: tse TR 3500–4500, TE 100–120)
- Slice thickness: 4 mm
- Interslice interval: 1.0–1.25
- Phase: AP
- Saturators: (a) perpendicular to the slices, block saturates the region in front of the spine; (b) transverse over the slices (reduces cerebrospinal fluid pulsation)
2. *Sagittal sequence*
- T1 (example: SE, TR 450–600, TE 12–25)
- Slice thickness, interval and saturation as in basic sequence 1 (see above)

3. *Transverse sequence* (through the region of interest)
–   T2 (example: gradient echo 1.5 T: TR 850, TE 26, pulse angle 30°; 0.5 T: TR 55, TE 27, pulse angle 6°)
–   Slice thickness: 4 mm
–   Interslice interval: 1.0
–   Saturation: perpendicular (coronal) to the slices, block saturates the region in front of the spine; transverse over (or also under) the slices
4. *Coronal sequence:* as in basic sequence 1 (see above)
Possible 5th *transverse sequence* (through the region of interest as in sequence 3)
–   T1 (example: tse TR 500–700, TE 10–25)
6. *Sagittal sequence* T1: as in sequence 2, but after contrast administration

MRI of the Lumbar Spine (or Thoracic Spine)

▨ Patient Preparation

– Patient should visit the rest room before the examination
– Patient should be given information about the procedure, with particular mention of how to avoid motion artifacts (comfortable positioning, no pain)
– Ear protection (e.g. ear plugs) should be offered
– Any metal items should be removed (dentures, hearing aids, hairpins, piercing, etc.)
– An indwelling catheter may be placed (e.g., if tumor, multiple sclerosis, spondylodiskitis, or abscess need to be investigated)

▲ Positioning

– Supine, spinal coil, cushions placed under the legs and immobilized if needed, arms in obese patients placed above head, otherwise alongside the body

Sequences

– Scout: sagittal and coronal (best with three levels)
1. *Sagittal sequence* (mark on coronal scout view, with as many slices as are necessary to fully image the spine)
– T2 (example: tse TR 3000–3500, TE 100–120)
– Slice thickness: 4 mm
– Interslice interval: 1.0
– Phase: FH, but then 100% oversampling or PA (thoracic spine)
– Saturation: (a) coronal, block saturates area in front of the spine (aorta, intestines, breathing artifacts); possibly (b) coronal, saturation of the dorsal fatty tissue

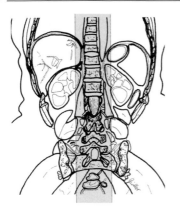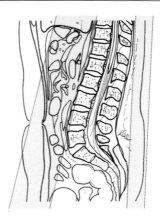

Sagittal lumbar spine, sequence 1

2. *Sagittal sequence* (as sequence 1)
– Protons (example: tse, example: TR 1200–1700, TE 12–20) or T1 (example: se TR 450–600, TE 12–25)
– Phase: AP
– Slice thickness, interval, and saturation as in sequence 1
– Or sequence 1 + 2: sagittal double echo, otherwise as in sequence 1
3. *Transverse sequence:* parallel to the corresponding vertebral surfaces (each segment usually has to be adjusted individually; if there are no abnormalities, routinely record the last three segments; *caution:* dorsal overlapping of slices should be outside the spinous processes if possible)
– Protons (example: tse TR 1700, TE 12) or T2 (example: gradient echo 1.5 T: TR 850, TE 26, pulse angle 30°; 0.5 T: TR 55, TE 27, pulse angle 6°)
– Slice thickness: 3–4 mm
– Interslice interval: 1.0
– Phase-encoding direction: PA
– Saturation: perpendicular (coronal) to the slices; block saturates area in front of the spine

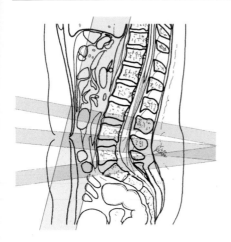

Transverse lumbar spine, parallel to the corresponding vertebral surfaces, sequence 3

4. *Coronal sequence*
– T2 (tse with higher turbo factor—e.g., TR 3000, TE 140)
– Slice thickness: 6 mm
– Interslice interval: 1.0
– Saturation: no

! Tips & Tricks

– In patients with more rounded backs, place cushions under the back; in those with additional cervical symptoms, the head can be raised and cushioned
– If there is severe scoliosis, ensure that enough slices are used to include the lateral areas
– Adjustment aids (thoracic spine): centering at about 3 FB below the throat (up to the mid-sternum)
– Adjustment aids (lumbar spine): centering on the anterior superior iliac spine or iliac crest (in large patients)

Examination after Intervertebral Disk Surgery in the Lumbar Spine

Patient Preparation

– An indwelling catheter with an extension tube should be placed

Sequences

1. *Sagittal sequence* T2 (see above, basic sequence 1)
2. *Sagittal sequence* protons (see above, basic sequence 2)
3. *Transverse sequence* (parallel to the corresponding vertebral surfaces)
– T1 (example: SE, TR 450–600, TE 12–25)
– Slice thickness: 4 mm
– Interslice interval: 1.0–1.2
– Saturation: (a) perpendicular (coronal) to the slices; block saturates area in front of the spine; (b) transverse (parallel to the slices) over the slice block; and (c) transverse (parallel to the slices) under the slice block
4. *Transverse sequence:* exactly as in sequence 3, but after contrast administration (e. g., Gd-DTPA)

Possible *5th sagittal sequence* T1: as above, but after contrast administration

Suspected Tumor, Suspected Spondylodiskitis, Abscess

Patient Preparation

– An indwelling catheter with an extension tube should be placed

1. *Sagittal sequence,* T2 sagittal (see above, basic sequence 1)
2. *Sagittal sequence* (as sequence 1)
– T1 (example: se, TR 450–600, TE 12–25)
– Slice thickness, interval and saturation as in sequence 1
3. *Transverse sequence* (through the region of interest)
– T1 (example: tse TR 500, TE 15)
– Slice thickness: 4 mm
– Interslice interval: 1.0
– Saturation: perpendicular (coronal) to the slices, block saturates the area in front of the spine
4. *Transverse sequence* T1: as sequence 3, but after contrast administration
5. *Sagittal sequence* T1: as sequence 2, but after contrast administration (e. g., Gd-DTPA)

Trauma, Suspected Fracture

See section on MRI of the Cervical Spine, above.

Sacroiliac Joint

1. *Sagittal sequence* T2 (example: tse TR 2500–4000, TE 100–130)
   – Slice thickness: 6 mm
   – Interslice interval: 1.0
   – Saturation: (a) transverse over the slices to saturate vessels; (b) coronal, ventral over the subcutaneous fatty tissue and bowel

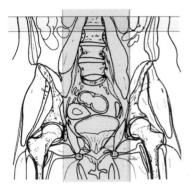
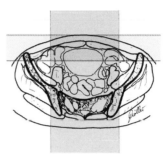

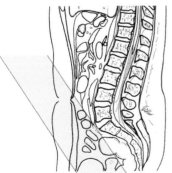

Sagittal sacroiliac joint, sequence 1

2. *Paracoronal sequence* T2 parallel to the sacrum (mark on the mid-sagittal slice), fat-saturated (example: tse TR 2500–4000, TE 100–120)
   – or turbo inversion recovery (TIRM) or spectral presaturation with inversion recovery (SPIR) (example: 1.5 T: TR 6500, TE [14] 30–60, TI 140, pulse angle 180°; 0.5 T: TR 2500, TE 60, TI 100)

- Slice thickness: 4–6 mm
- Interslice interval: 1.0–1.2
- Saturation: coronal, ventral over the slices

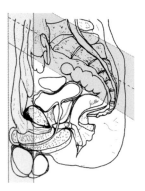

Paracoronal sacroiliac joint,
parallel to the sacrum, sequence 2

3. *Paracoronal sequence:* as sequence 2, but T1 (example: se TR 450–600, TE 12–25)

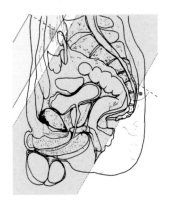

Paratransverse sacroiliac joint, sequence 3

4. *Paratransverse sequence* T1 (example: se TR 500–700, TE 12–25)
- Slice thickness: 4–6 mm
- Interslice interval: 1.3–1.5
- Two saturators: (a) ventral, coronal (perpendicular to the slices) over the abdominal fatty tissue; and (b) transverse over the slices for vascular saturation

MRI of the Chest

■ Patient Preparation

- Patient should visit the rest room before the examination
- Patient should be given information about the procedure
- All clothes except underwear should be removed
- Any metal items should be removed (hearing aids, hairpins, piercing, necklaces, etc.)

▲ Positioning

- Supine, body array coil or body coil, cushions placed under the legs, headphones worn if needed

Sequences

- Scout: transverse and sagittal (best with three levels)
1. *Coronal sequence*
- T2 (1.5 T: tse, breath-holding, example: TR 3000–4000, TE 130–140, pulse angle 180°; 0.5 T: tse, breath-triggered, example: TR 1666 or 2500 [2–3 respiration cycles], TE 100, pulse angle 90°)
- Slice thickness: 8 mm
- Interslice interval: 1.0
- Phase-encoding direction: FH
- Saturation: no

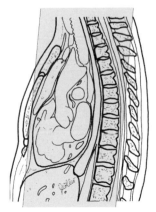
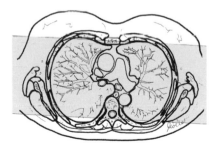

Coronal thorax, sequence 1

2. *Transverse sequence*
- T2, whole lung from the apex to the costophrenic angle (1.5 T: tse, breath-holding, example: TR 3000–4000, TE 130–140, pulse angle 180°; 0.5 T: tse, breath-triggered, example: TR 1666 or 2500 [2–3 respiration cycles], TE 100, pulse angle 90°)
- Slice thickness: 8 mm
- Interslice interval: 1.0
- Phase-encoding direction: AP
- Saturation: ventral (coronal) to saturate the subcutaneous fatty tissue

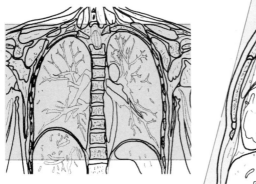 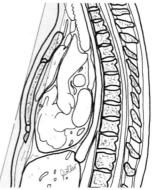

Transverse thorax, sequence 2

3. *Transverse sequence* T1, otherwise as in sequence 1
- T1 (example: 1.5 T, breath-holding, gradient echo (FLASH) TR 120–140, TE 4, pulse angle 60°; 0.5 T: breath-compensated, TR 500–600, TE 10, pulse angle 90°)

! Tips & Tricks
- Electrocardiographic (ECG) triggering can be used
- With breath triggering, the patient should be asked to breathe regularly
- When a chest wall tumor is being investigated, the patient should be placed on the tumor side if appropriate (reduces motion artifacts in this area)

Chest with Gd-DTPA

▦ **Patient Preparation**
– Place an indwelling catheter

Sequences

1. *Coronal sequence:* T2 as above, basic sequence 1
2. *Transverse sequence:* T2 as above, basic sequence 2
3. *Transverse sequence:* T1 as above, basic sequence 3
4. *Transverse sequence:* T1 as sequence 3 but after Gd-DTPA administration
Possible *5th coronal sequence:* T1 (as above) after Gd-DTPA administration

Magnetic Resonance Imaging

Upper Abdominal MRI (Liver)

▦ Patient Preparation

– Patient should visit the rest room before the examination
– Patient should be given information about the procedure
– All clothes except underwear should be removed
– Any metal items should be removed (hearing aids, hairpins, piercing, etc.)

▲ Positioning

– Supine, body array coil or body coil, cushions placed under the legs, head-phones worn if needed

Sequences

– Scout: coronal and sagittal, with three levels if possible
1. *Transverse sequence*
– T2 from the dome of the liver to the aortic bifurcation (1.5 T: tse, breath-holding, example: TR 3000–4000, TE 130–140, pulse angle 180°; 0.5 T: tse, breath-triggered, example: TR 1666 or 2500 [2–3 respiration cycles], TE 100, pulse angle 90°)
– Slice thickness: 8 mm
– Interslice interval: 1.0
– Phase-encoding direction: AP
– Saturation: transverse (parallel) to the slices to saturate the vessels, and ventral (coronal) to saturate the subcutaneous fatty tissue

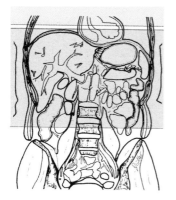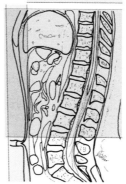

Transverse liver/upper abdomen, sequence 1

2. *Transverse sequence*
- T1 otherwise as in sequence 1 (example: 1.5 T, breath-holding: gradient echo [FLASH], TR 120–140, TE 4, pulse angle 60°; or breath-holding SE [1 T], TR 300, repeated 3–4 times until the organ is fully imaged. 0.5 T: breath-compensated, TR 500–600, TE 10, pulse angle 90°)

3. *Coronal sequence*
- T2 (1.5 T: tse, breath-holding, example: TR 3000–4000, TE 130–140, pulse angle 180°; 0.5 T: tse, breath-triggered, example: TR 1900–2300, TE 100, pulse angle 90°)
- Slice thickness: 8 mm
- Interslice interval: 1.0
- Phase-encoding direction: RL
- Saturation: transverse over the slices for vascular saturation

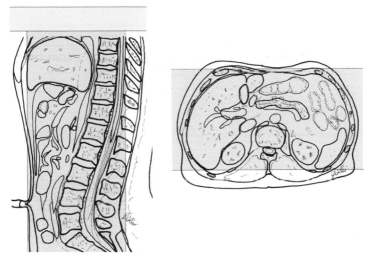

Coronal liver/upper abdomen, sequence 3

❗ Tips & Tricks

- Intravenous hyoscine butylbromide (Buscopan) can be used to reduce bowel motility
- Bowel contrast (e.g., Abdoscan)

Liver after Superparamagnetic Contrast (Endorem)

1. *Transverse sequence:* T2 as in basic sequence 1
2. *Transverse sequence:* T1 as in basic sequence 1

Remove the patient from the device. Inject the contrast medium (Endorem) by intravenous infusion.

Approx. 60–90 min after the start of the injection:

3. *Transverse sequence:* T2 as above, but after Endorem administration
4. *Transverse sequence:* T1 as above, but after Endorem administration
5. *Coronal sequence:* T2 as above, but after Endorem administration

Liver with Gd-DTPA

■ **Patient Preparation**

– Place an indwelling catheter

Sequences

1. *Transverse sequence:* T2 as in basic sequence 1
3. *Transverse sequence:* T1 as in basic sequence 1
3. *Transverse sequence:* T1 as above, but after Gd-DTPA administration

Possible *3rd–8th transverse sequences:* T1 dynamic
Possible *9th transverse sequence:* T1 as late image approx. 5 min post-injection

Magnetic Resonance Imaging

Biliary Tract

Paracoronal sequence (adjusted to the course of the common bile duct = approx. 0–30° to the horizontal, mark on the axial image)

- T2, fat-saturated (example: 1.5 T: HASTE TR 11.9, TE 95, pulse angle 150°; 0.5 T: (3D IR TSE, breath-triggered), TR 1666 or 2500, TE 700, TI 90, slice thickness 4 mm with 50% overlap = 2 mm, then MIP analysis)
  or single-slice technique:
- T2, fat-saturated with high TE (example: TR 2800, TE 1100, pulse angle 150°, slice thickness 70 mm—no MIP analysis necessary)
- FOV large (at least 35 cm, to avoid wrap-around artifacts)

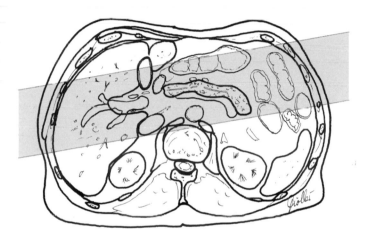

Paracoronal biliary tract

Magnetic Resonance Imaging

MRI of the Pelvis

■ Patient Preparation

– Patient should visit the rest room before the examination
– Patient should be given information about the procedure and should be offered ear protection (e.g. ear plugs)
– All clothes except underwear should be removed
– Any metal items should be removed (hearing aids, hairpins, piercing, etc.)
– Depending on the issue being investigated, the patient should drink one bag of oral contrast (e.g., Abdoscan) 1 h before the examination
– An indwelling catheter may be placed

▲ Positioning

– Supine, body array coil or body coil, cushions placed under the legs

Sequences

– Scout: sagittal and transverse (three levels if possible)
1. *Transverse sequence:*
– T2, possibly fat-saturated (example: tse TR 2500–4500, TE 100–130)
– Slice thickness: 8 mm
– Interslice interval: 1–1.3
– Phase-encoding direction: AP
– Saturation: (a) transverse (parallel) over the slices for vascular saturation; (b) ventral, coronal (perpendicular to the slices) over the abdominal fatty tissue

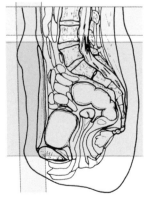 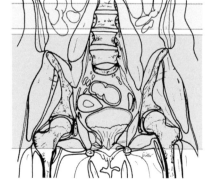

Transverse pelvis, sequence 1

2. *Transverse sequence:*
- T1 (example: se TR: 450–600, TE 12–25)
- Slice thickness: 8 mm
- Interslice interval: 1.3
- Phase-encoding direction: AP
- Saturation: (a) ventral, coronal (perpendicular to the slices) over the abdominal fatty tissue; (b) transverse over the slices for vascular saturation
3. *Coronal sequence:*
- T2 (example: tse TR 2500–4500, TE 100–130)
- Slice thickness: 5 6 mm
- Interslice interval: 1.3
- Phase-encoding direction: HF
- Saturation: transverse over the slices for vascular saturation

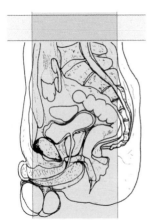
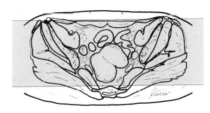

Coronal pelvis, sequence 3

Possible 4th transverse sequence: T1 as in sequence 2, but after contrast administration (Gd-DTPA)

❗ Tips & Tricks
....
- Intravenous Buscopan can be administered to reduce bowel motility
- An "abdominal bandage" can be applied to limit respiratory excursions

Uterus, Vagina, Bladder

1. *Transverse sequence:* T2 (as in basic sequence 1 above)
2. *Transverse sequence:* T1 (as in basic sequence 2 above)
3. *Coronal sequence:* (possible pelvic inclination should be taken into consideration)
– Turbo inversion recovery (TIRM) or short tau inversion recovery (STIR) (example: 1.5 T: TR 6500, TE 14, TI 140, pulse angle 90°; 0.5 T: TR 1800, TE [14] 30–60, TI 100, pulse angle 90°) or fat-saturated T2 (example: tse TR 2500–4000, TE 100–120)
– Slice thickness: 4 mm
– Interslice interval: 1.0
– Saturation: transverse over the slices for vascular saturation

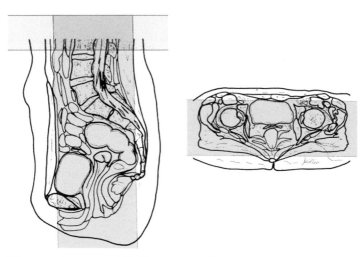

Uterus, vagina, coronal bladder, sequence 3

4. *Sagittal sequence:*
– T2 (example: tse TR 2500–3500, TE 100–130)
– Slice thickness: 8 mm
– Interslice interval: 1.0

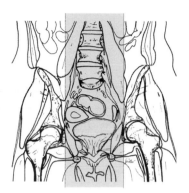 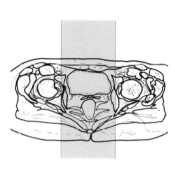

Uterus, vagina, sagittal bladder, sequence 4

Prostate

Patient Preparation
....
– Endorectal capsule if needed
1. *Transverse sequence:* over the pelvic floor (mark on sagittal scout view)
– T2, 512 (or 256) matrix (example: tse TR 2500–4000, TE 100–130)
– Slice thickness: 3–4 mm
– Interslice interval: 1.0
– FOV: small (e.g., 250 mm; with 512 matrix, carry out 4–6 mean calculations due to the signal-to-noise ratio)
– Phase: AP
– Two saturations: (a) transverse (parallel) over the slices for vascular saturation; (b) ventral, coronal (at right angles to the slices) over the abdominal fatty tissue

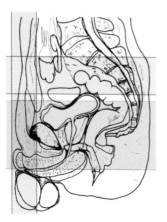

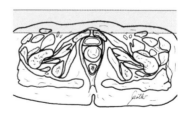

Transverse prostate over the pelvic floor, sequence 1

2. *Coronal sequence:*
   – T2, 512 (or 256) matrix (example: tse TR 2500–4000, TE 100–130)
   – Slice thickness: 3 mm
   – Interslice interval: 1.0
   – FOV: small (e.g., 250 mm; with 512 matrix, carry out 4–6 mean calculations)
   – Phase: LR
   – Saturation: transverse (parallel) over the slices for vascular saturation

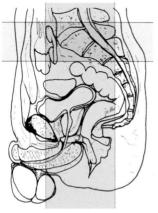

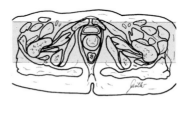

Coronal prostate, sequence 2

3. *Transverse sequence:*
- T1, 512 matrix (example: se TR 500–700, TE 12–25)
- Slice thickness: 3 mm
- Interslice interval: 1.0
- Phase: AP
- Saturations: (a) ventral, coronal (at right angles to the slices) over the abdominal fatty tissue; (b) transverse over the slices for vascular saturation

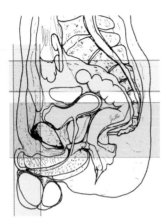

Transverse prostate, sequence 3

4. *Transverse sequence:*
- T1 as in sequence 2, but after contrast administration (Gd-DTPA)

Possible *5th sequence, coronal or sagittal* over the prostate:
- T1, 512 matrix (TR 500–700, TE 12–25)
- Slice thickness: 3 mm
- Interslice interval: 1.0
- Phase: AP
- Saturation: transverse over the slices for vascular saturation

MRI of the Shoulder

■ Patient Preparation

- Patient should visit the rest room before the examination
- Patient should be given information about the procedure and should be offered ear protection (e.g. ear plugs)
- All clothes except underwear should be removed
- Any metal items should be removed (hearing aids, hairpins, piercing, necklaces, etc.)
- Depending on the issue being investigated, the patient should drink one bag of oral contrast (e. g., Abdoscan) 1 h before the examination
- An indwelling catheter may be placed

▲ Positioning

- Supine, shoulder coil (oval surface coil, flexible coil), arm in neutral position or supination, cushions placed under the legs

Sequences

- Scout: axial and coronal
1. *Transverse sequence:*
- T2 (tse, example: TR 2500–4500, TE 100–130 or gradient echo [to display the labrum: FLASH, TR 600–700, TE 11, phase angle 60°])
- Slice thickness: 4 mm
- Interslice interval: 1.2
- Saturation: no

2. *Paracoronal sequence* (parallel to the course of the supraspinatus muscle on the transverse slice):
- T2 fat-saturated (example: tse TR 2500–4000, TE 100–120 or STIR: TR 2200, TE 60, TI 100, phase angle 90°)
- Slice thickness: 4 mm
- Interslice interval: 1.0
- Saturation: parasagittal, oblique to the slice over the lung

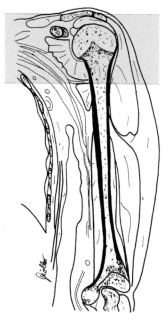

Transverse shoulder, sequence 1

Paracoronal shoulder, sequence 2

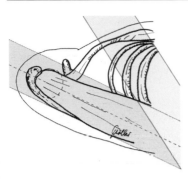

3. *Paracoronal sequence:*
– As in sequence 2, but T1-weighted (example: 1.5 T: TR 500–600, TE 12, phase angle 90°; 0.5 T: TR 500–600, TE 10–17, phase angle 90°)
4. *Presagittal sequence* (at right angles to sequence 2 over the joint or parallel to the socket)
– T1 (example: TR 500–600, TE 10–20)
– Slice thickness: 4 mm
– Interslice interval: 1.0
– Saturation: over the lung

Parasagittal shoulder, sequence 4

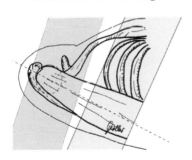

❗ Tips & Tricks
– Positioning: immobilize the coil laterally with sandbags. Place sandbags or a belt over the lower arm in supination (if this is difficult, it is better to use a neutral position)
– Raise the patient slightly (approx. 45°) to the contralateral side and provide appropriate cushions to prevent imaging artifacts ("magic angle effects")

Indirect Arthrography of the Shoulder (e. g., for Labrum Diagnosis)

▉ Patient Preparation
....

– 30 min before the examination, give the patient an intravenous injection of 0.2 mmol/kg body weight (ca. 10 mL) Gd-DTPA. Have the patient move the shoulder
1. *Transverse sequence:*
– T1 fat-saturated (example: se TR 450–700, TE 12–25)
– Slice thickness: 4 mm
– Interslice interval: 1.2
– Saturation: no
2. *Paracoronal sequence:*
– T2 (as sequence 2)
3. *Paracoronal sequence:*
– T1 fat-saturated (otherwise as in sequence 3)
4. *Parasagittal sequence:*
– T1 fat-saturated (otherwise as in sequence 4)

Magnetic Resonance Imaging

MRI of the Hip

▩ Patient Preparation

- Patient should visit the rest room before the examination
- Patient should be given information about the procedure and should be offered ear protection (e.g. ear plugs)
- All clothes except underwear should be removed
- Any metal items should be removed (hearing aids, hairpins, piercing, etc.)

▲ Positioning

- Supine, body array coil (body coil), cushions placed under the legs

Sequences

- Scout: transverse and coronal
1. *Coronal sequence* over the femoral heads (possible pelvic inclination should be taken into consideration)
- Turbo inversion recovery (TIRM) or short tau inversion recovery (STIR) (example: 1.5 T: TR 6500, TE [14], TI 140, pulse angle 180°; 0.5 T: TR 1800, TE 60, TI 100, pulse angle 90°) or fat-saturated (14) 30–60 T2 (example: tse TR 2500–4000, TE 100–120)
- Slice thickness: 4 mm
- Interslice interval: 1.0
- Phase-encoding gradient: RL
- Saturation: transverse over the slices for vascular saturation

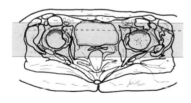

Coronal hip over femoral head, sequence 1

2. *Coronal sequence* over the femoral heads (possible pelvic inclination should be taken into consideration)
- T1 (example: se TR 450–600, TE 12–25)
- Slice thickness: 4–6 mm
- Interslice interval: 1.0
- Phase-encoding gradient: RL
- Saturation: transverse over the slices for vascular saturation
3. *Transverse sequence* over the femoral heads and acetabula (caudad up to the end of the greater trochanter)

- T2 (example: tse TR 2500–4000, TE 100–120)
- Slice thickness: 8 mm
- Interslice interval: 1.0
- Saturation: transverse (parallel) over the slices for vascular saturation

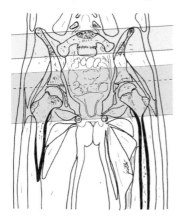

Transverse hip over femoral head and acetabulum, sequence 3

4. *Sagittal sequence* (over both femoral heads)
- T1 (example: TR 500–600, TE 10–25)
- Slice thickness: 6–8 mm
- Interslice interval: 1.0
- Saturation: transverse

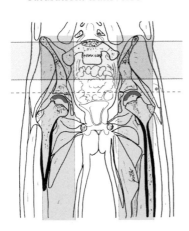
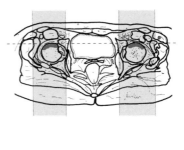

Sagittal hip over both femoral heads, sequence 4

❗ Tips & Tricks

– Adjustment aids: centering on the anterior inferior iliac spine
– When there are vascular artifacts from the iliac vessels, the phase-encoding gradient can be rotated in the head–feet direction (with oversampling to prevent wrap-around artifacts)

MRI of the Knee

▨ Patient Preparation

– Patient should visit the rest room before the examination
– Patient should be given information about the procedure and should be offered ear protection (e.g. ear plugs)
– All clothes except underwear should be removed
– Any metal items should be removed (hearing aids, hairpins, piercing, watch, etc.)

▲ Positioning

– Supine, 10–15° external rotation, knee immobilized in the coil, other leg comfortably cushioned
– Articular cavity in the center of the coil

Sequences

– Scout: sagittal and transverse (best with three levels)

1. *Coronal sequence:*
– Turbo inversion recovery (TIRM) or spectral presaturation with inversion recovery (SPIR) (example: 1.5 T: TR 6500, TE [14] 30–60, TI 140, pulse angle 180°; 0.5 T: TR 2000, TE 40, TI 40, pulse angle 90°) or fat-saturated T2 (example: tse TR 2500–4000, TE 100–120)
– Slice thickness: 3 mm
– Interslice interval: 1.0
– Saturation: no

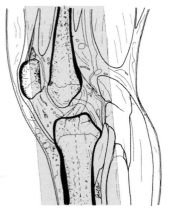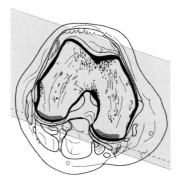

Coronal knee, sequence 1

2. *Sagittal sequence* (= perpendicular to 1)
- 3D gradient echo (example: 1.5 T: DESS, TR 25, TE 9, phase angle 35°; 0.5 T: FFE, TR shortest possible [e.g., 95], TE 27, phase angle 25°)
- Block thickness: 100–120 mm (effective thickness approx. 1.5 mm)
- Partitions: 64
- Saturation: transverse over the slices

Alternative sagittal sequence 2 (= perpendicular to 1)
- T2, fat-saturated (example: tse TR 2500–4000, TE 100–120)
- Slice thickness: 3 mm
- Interslice interval: 1.0
- Saturation: transverse over the slices

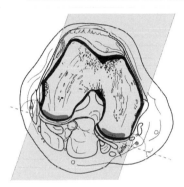

Sagittal knee, sequence 2

3. *Transverse sequence:*
- T2 (example: tse TR 2500–400, TE 100–120)
- Slice thickness: 3 mm
- Interslice interval: 1.0
- Saturation: transverse over the slices (parallel over the slices)

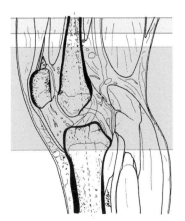

Transverse knee, sequence 3

Magnetic Resonance Imaging

4. *Sagittal* or *coronal* sequence:
- T1 (example: se TR 450–600, TE 12–25 or STIR: TR 2200, TE 32, phase angle 90°)
- Slice thickness: 3–6 mm
- Interslice interval: 1.2
- Saturation: transverse over the slices

! Tips & Tricks
- Provide good cushioning underneath the knee

Knee Examination with Gadolinium
(e. g., for Investigating Tumor, Osteochondritis Dissecans)

▨ Patient Preparation
- An indwelling catheter with an extension tube should be placed

Sequences
1. *Coronal sequence* TIRM or SPIR (see above, basic sequence 1)
2. *Sagittal sequence* 3D GE (see above, basic sequence 2)
3. *Coronal sequence:*
- T1 (example: se TR 450–700, TE 12–25)
- Slice thickness: 6 mm
- Interslice interval: 1.2
- Saturation: no
4. Coronal sequence:
- As sequence 3, but after contrast administration (Gd-DTPA, 0.1 mL/kg body weight)
5. *Transverse sequence:*
- T1 (example: se TR 500–700, TE 12–25)
- Slice thickness: 4–6 mm
- Interslice interval: 1.2
- Saturation: transverse, proximal to the slices (or parallel to the slices)

AP
Anteroposterior
CC
Craniocaudal
CISS
Constructive interference in steady state
CT
Computed tomography
DESS
Double-echo steady state
DSA
Digital subtraction angiography
ECG
Electrocardiography
FB
Fingerbreadth
FFE
Fast field echo
FH
Foot to head (phase-encoding direction)
FLAIR
Fluid-attenuated inversion recovery
FLASH
Fast low-angle shot
FOV
Field of view
GE
Gradient echo
HASTE
half-Fourier acquisition single-shot turbo spin echo
HF
Head to foot (phase-encoding direction)
HU
Hounsfield unit
IR
Inversion recovery
LAO
Left anterior oblique
LM
Lateromedial
LR
Left to right (phase-encoding direction)
MIP
Maximum-intensity projection
ML
Mediolateral
MLO
Mediolateral oblique

MPR
Multiplanar reconstruction
MRI
Magnetic resonance imaging
N
Newton
PA
Posteroanterior
PNL
Pectoral–nipple line
PT
Prothrombin time
PTT
Partial thromboplastin time
RAO
Right anterior oblique
RL
Right to left (phase-encoding direction)
ROI
Region of interest
SC
Sensitivity class
SE
Spin echo
SID
Source-to-image receptor distance
SPIR
Spectral presaturation with inversion recovery
STIR
Short tau inversion recovery
Topo
Topogram
TE
Echo time
TI
Inversion time
TIR
Turbo inversion recovery
TIRM
Turbo inversion recovery measurement
TR
Repetition time
VTR
Videotape recording
WL
Window level
WW
Window width

3D measurement
Volume measurement; an imaging technique in which, during each stimulating pulse, the entire volume of interest is stimulated instead of a single slice

Abduction
Movement away from the body

Adduction
Movement toward the body

Anteflexion
Bending forward

Anterior
In front

Anteroposterior (AP)
From the front toward the back

Articulation
Joint

Boxer position
See LAO (second oblique diameter)

Bucky (diffuse radiation screen)
A moving grid that prevents diffuse radiation arising in the object

Caudal
Downward

Caudocranial
From below to above

Caudodorsal
From below (obliquely) toward the back

Caudomedial
From below (obliquely) toward the middle

Central ray
The ray that emerges from the center of the X-ray tube and passes through the center of the radiation discharge window perpendicular to the axis of the tube

Craniocaudal
From above to below

Craniolateral
From above (obliquely) to the side

Cranioventral
From above (obliquely) to the front

Detector
Usually a flat detector. Converts radiation directly into a digital image. Is used instead of traditional X-ray cassettes and is integrated into the radiography table

Distal
Away from (the center of) the body

Dorsal
Toward the back

Dorsoplantar
From the back of the foot to the sole

Dorsoventral
From the back to the front

Dorsovolar
From the back of the hand to the palm

Expiration
Breathing out

Eye–ear line
The reference line between the lateral corner of the eye and the center of the auditory canal

Fencer position
See RAO (first oblique diameter)

FFE
Fast field echo = fast imaging with steady precession (FISP) = gradient echo (GE) = gradient-recalled acquisition of steady state (GRASS) = gradient-recalled echo (GRE): gradient echo measurement in which the transverse and longitudinal magnetization contribute to the image. The contrast is a ratio of T1 to T2*

FISP
See FFE

FLAIR
Fluid-attenuated inversion recovery; see TIRM

FLASH
Fast low-angle shot. T1-FFE = spoiled GRASS (SPGR): at equilibrium, only the longitudinal magnetization is used and transverse magnetization is destroyed by the "spoiler." T1-weighted or T2*-weighted contrast can be set

Flow compensation
Method of avoiding movement-related signal loss and incorrect registration

FOV
Field of view: the area of a slice that is displayed

Frontal
Toward the forehead

Gap
Gap between two slice boundaries (1.1 = 10% gap = a gap of 0.8 mm at a slice thickness of 8 mm)

Gd-DTPA
Gadolinium diethylenetriaminepenta-acetic acid complex, a gadolinium chelate; (positive) contrast medium that shortens T1 (e.g., Magnevist)

German horizontal
The reference line between the lower edge of the eye and the upper external auditory canal

Gradient echo (GE)
Gradient-recalled echo (GRE): see FFE

Gradual sheet
Compensation sheet

Gray
Unit of energy dosage (formerly rad; 1 rad = 0.01 Gy)

Humeroulnar
From the upper arm obliquely toward the ulna

Image display device
Screen or monitor

Image receiver
Anything that converts the radiation into an image: a detector, such as the traditional film

Image receiver dosage
Permissible threshold values apply to film sheet systems and also in digital radiography

Imaging system
Used instead of the film sheet system; includes digital systems

Inversion recovery (IR)
A pulse sequence in which the magnetization is initially inverted by a 180° pulse before the stimulation pulses for signal recording. The waiting time between the inversion pulse and the 90° pulse is called the inversion time (TI), and it determines the extent of the T1 weighting. Can be used for T1-weighted images, but is also used for fat suppression (with a short T1: STIR) or for water suppression (with a long T1: FLAIR, TIRM)

LAO
Left anterior oblique (front left oblique), second oblique diameter

Laterodorsal
From the side (obliquely) toward the back

Lateroventral
From the side (obliquely) toward the front

Lordosis
Curvature of the spine toward the front

Matrix
Image matrix: determines the number of image points on each edge of the image—e.g., 128, 256, or 512 pixels

Maximum intensity projection (MIP)
A reconstruction method in which the strong signals are filtered out and projected on one level

Mediosagittal
In the center of the long axis of the body

ML
Mediolateral

MLO
Mediolateral oblique

Occipital
Toward the back of the head

Occipitomental
From the back of the head toward the chin

Occipitonasal
From the back of the head towards the nose

Occipito-orbital
From the back of the head toward the orbit (cavity containing the eyeball)

Oversampling
Fold-over suppression; a method of avoiding folding artefacts

Phase
Fold-over direction = phase encoding gradient = folding direction = preparation direction. Folding artifacts (aliasing) and pulsation artefacts appear in the direction of the phase-coded gradient

Phase angle
Synonymous with pulse angle (PA): the stimulation angle of the magnetization. Typically selected as < 90° in GE sequences; its effect determines the extent of T1 weighting and therefore always has to be stated in GE sequences. In spin echo measurements, the angle is usually 90°

Philtrum
Median groove in the upper lip

Pitch factor
Ratio of the table advancement per tube rotation to the slice thickness

Plantar
Toward the sole of the foot

Posteroanterior (PA)
From the back toward the front

Pronation
Rotating inward

Proton density–weighted
Pulse sequence with short TE and long TR, so that the images are neither T1-weighted nor T2-weighted

Proximal
Near the body, toward the middle of the body

Radial
Toward the radius

Radioulnar
From the radius toward the ulna

RAO
Right anterior oblique (front right oblique), second oblique diameter

Reclination
Bending backward

Reconstruction index
Width of the slices subsequently calculated from the CT spiral data set

Retroflexion
See Reclination

Saturation
Excitation of spins—e.g., with a fast sequence of pulses, so that T1 relaxation is suppressed and is therefore left unphased on the x–y level. Saturated spins are not available for imaging in immediately subsequent pulse sequences and therefore do not contribute to the image signal

Scoliosis
Curvature of the spine toward the side

Scout
Planning scan = localizer = survey. A fast initial MR measurement for positional orientation and planning of diagnostic imaging

SE
Spin echo measurement: imaging procedure in which the spins producing an echo are refocused by a 180° pulse. In the conventional pulse sequence, one or more echoes per stimulation pulse are read out with a fixed phase coding

Sensitivity class
Sensitivity of the film sheet system (sensitivity class 100 corresponds to a dosage requirement of 10 µGy for an optical density [D = 1] higher than the veil or base)

SPIR
Spectral presaturation with inversion recovery. A frequency-selective method of fat suppression in which the fat signal is stimulated by frequency-selective saturation or inversion pulses in such a way that it does not contribute to the image intensity

STIR
Short tau inversion recovery. An inversion recovery pulse sequence with a short inversion time (TI) for suppression of the fat signal. All signals with short T1 times, like those of fat, are suppressed, and the technique is therefore not generally indicated after contrast administration

Submental
Under the chin

T1-FFE
See FLASH

T1-weighted
T1w: image with a short repetition time (TR) and short echo time (TE). Tissues with short T1 values are bright in T1w images; tissues with long T1 values are dark in T1w images

T2-weighted
T2w: an image with a long repetition time (TR) and long echo time (TE). Tissues with short T2 values are dark on T2w images; tissue with long T2 values are bright on T2w images

TE
Echo time: the time between stimulation and the center of the signal read-out

Tesla (T)
The strength of the magnetic field. The most widely used devices have 0.5 T, 1.0 T, and 1.5 T

TI
Inversion time: the waiting time between the inversion pulse and the 90° pulse in inversion recovery pulse sequences

TIRM
Turbo inversion recovery measurement = (turbo-) fluid-attenuated inversion recovery (FLAIR). Measurement with a long inversion time (TI) to suppress the water signal in T2-weighted stimulation pulses

TR
Repetition time. The interval between two successive stimulation pulses

TSE
Turbo spin echo. A fast spin echo measurement, with a multiple echo sequence within a single TR time with different phase encodings per echo

Turbo factor
The number of multiple echoes and thus shortening of the measuring time in comparison with the traditional sequence

Ulnohumeral
From the ulna (obliquely) toward the upper arm

Ulnoradial
From the ulna toward the radius

Ventrodorsal
From the abdomen toward the back

Volar
Toward the palm

Becht S, Bittner RC, Ohmstede A, Pfeiffer A, Rossdeutscher R. Lehrbuch der röntgendiagnostischen Einstelltechnik. Berlin: Springer, 2007.

Bernau A. Orthopädische Röntgendiagnostik—Einstelltechnik. Munich: Urban & Schwarzenberg, 1982.

Biederer JJ, Wildberger E, Reuter M, Bolte H, Fink C, Tuengerthal S, et al. Protokollempfehlungen für die Computertomographie der Lunge. Röfo 2008; 180:471–9.

Bittner RC, Hazim K, Helmig K. CT, EBT, MRT und Angiographie. Munich: Urban & Fischer, 2003.

Brusis T, Mödder U. HNO-Röntgenaufnahmetechnik. Berlin: Springer, 1984.

Dietze R, Köcher E. Physik und Praxis der Röntgenaufnahmetechnik. Jena: Fischer, 1982.

Fellner FA, Wallhör I, Grafinger Witt E, Schenk P. Mammakarzinom. Radiopraxis 2008;1:11–26.

General Medical Council, Federal Republic of Germany [*Bundesärztekammer*]. Leitlinie der Bundesärztekammer zur Qualitätssicherung in der Röntgendiagnostik [23 Nov 2007].

General Medical Council, Federal Republic of Germany [*Bundesärztekammer*]. Leitlinie der Bundesärztekammer zur Qualitätssicherung in der Computertomographie [23 Nov 2007].

General Medical Council, Federal Republic of Germany [*Bundesärztekammer*]. Leitlinien der Bundesärztekammer zur Qualitätssicherung in der Magnetresonanztomographie [29 Jan 1999]. Dt Ärztebl 2000; 97 (39):A2557–68.

Greenspan A. Orthopedic radiology: a practical approach, 2nd ed. New York: Raven Press, 1992.

Hip E. Röntgendiagnostik. In: Witt AN, ed. Orthopädie in Praxis und Klinik, vol. 2. Stuttgart: Thieme, 1980.

Hogarth B. Anatomisches Zeichnen leichtgemacht. Berlin: Taschen, 1991.

Husmann K, Mehrkens A, Hancken G. Radiologische Einstelltechnik. Berlin: Blackwell, 1995.

Jungbauer M. Röntgen-Einstelltechnik. 4 vols. Basel: Roche, 1979

Lichte-Wichmann M. Richtig eingestellt? Stuttgart: Thieme, 1993.

Lutz KC. Einstelltechniken in der Traumatologie. Stuttgart: Thieme, 1992.

Marcelis S, Seragini FC, Taylor JA, Huang GS, Park YH, Resnick D. Cervical spine: comparison of 45 degree and 55 degrees anteroposterior oblique radiographic projections. Radiology 1993;188:253–6.

Meschan I. Analyse der Röntgenbilder. Stuttgart: Enke, 1981.

Meschan I. Röntgenanatomie. Stuttgart: Enke, 1987.

Möller TB. MRT-Einstelltechnik. Stuttgart: Thieme, 2003.

Möller TB. Normal findings in radiography. New York: Thieme, 2001.

Möller TB, Reif E. Rezeptbuch radiologischer Verfahren. Berlin: Springer, 2002.

Möller TB, Reif E. Taschenatlas der Röntgenanatomie. Stuttgart: Thieme, 2006.

Möller TB, Reif E. Taschenatlas der Schnittbildanatomie. 3 vols. Stuttgart: Thieme, 2007.

Oetjen HW. Qualitätssicherung in der Computertomographie. Radiol Assist 1994;8.

Poppe H. Technik der Röntgendiagnostik, 3rd ed. Stuttgart: Thieme, 1972.

Ring B. Felsenbeinaufnahme nach Mayer. Radiol Assist 1991;5.

Ring-Baltruweit B. Schädel in 2 Ebenen. Radiol Assist 1993;7.

Rubins DK. Anatomie für Künstler. Ravensburg: Maier, 1970.

Sass U. Qualitätskriterien röntgendiagnostischer Untersuchungen. Radiol Assist 1991.

Tertilt A. Schwedenstatus. Radiol Assist 1990;45.

Wandt C. Ala- und Obturatum-Aufnahme. Radiol Assist 1992;6.

Wandt C. Axiale oder axilläre Schultergelenk-Aufnahme. Radiol Assist 1993; 7.

Wilhelm M. Vorschriftensammlung zum Vollzug der Röntgenverordnung. Munich: WRW-Verlag, 1995.